人体图典
奇妙身体说明书

**The Visual Dictionary
of the Human Body**

原著 ［加］QA国际
主译 王卫明 李 箭
审校 阎少华
译者 黄 轩 李瑞欣 李春辉 刘 佳 魏志亨

人民卫生出版社
·北 京·

内容简介

《人体图典：奇妙身体说明书》是一本人体各主要系统的图谱集，适合全家人阅读学习。本书汇集了人体各个部位的高清图像，并配有多种语言的术语解释。附加文字（简介和边栏）还给出了相关的补充资料，让您更好地了解本书所示人体各系统的特点和功能。

Introduction

The Visual Dictionary of the Human Body is a family atlas for exploration of the major systems of the human body. This book presents a collection of high-definition images of different parts of the body, linked to terms in several languages. Complementary texts (introductions and sidebars) offer additional information on the characteristics and functions of all systems shown.

标题

标题位于页面顶部，并同时给出中英对照的文字。如果一个标题连续出现在多个页面上，则在随后的页面上以灰度显示。

TITLE

Titles are located at the top of the page, with the other languages below. If a title continues on more than one page it is grayed out on subsequent pages.

主题

每个主题都对应着人体的各个系统和细分结构。主题以中英对照形式呈现在书中的每一页。

THEME

The themes correspond to the systems and divisions of the human body. They are presented on each page in the edition's main language.

图示

高度逼真的图示给相关的名词术语以视觉定义。

ILLUSTRATION

The extremely realistic illustrations contribute to the visual definition of the terms associated with them.

边栏

作为对正文的补充，边栏给出了一些不太寻常或令人新奇的内容。

SIDEBAR

Sidebars present unusual or surprising facts that complement the information in each section.

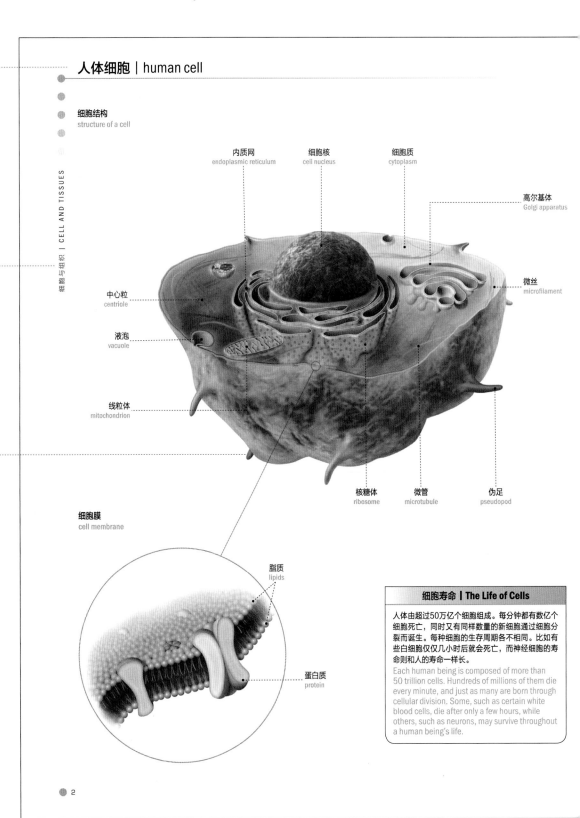

细胞与组织 | CELL AND TISSUES

人体细胞 | human cell

细胞结构
structure of a cell

内质网
endoplasmic reticulum

细胞核
cell nucleus

细胞质
cytoplasm

高尔基体
Golgi apparatus

微丝
microfilament

中心粒
centriole

液泡
vacuole

线粒体
mitochondrion

核糖体
ribosome

微管
microtubule

伪足
pseudopod

细胞膜
cell membrane

脂质
lipids

蛋白质
protein

细胞寿命 | The Life of Cells

人体由超过50万亿个细胞组成。每分钟都有数亿个细胞死亡，同时又有同样数量的新细胞通过细胞分裂而诞生。每种细胞的生存周期各不相同。比如有些白细胞仅仅几小时后就会死亡，而神经细胞的寿命则和人的寿命一样长。

Each human being is composed of more than 50 trillion cells. Hundreds of millions of them die every minute, and just as many are born through cellular division. Some, such as certain white blood cells, die after only a few hours, while others, such as neurons, may survive throughout a human being's life.

本书结构

本书共分14个主题。每个主题的开始都有一个对开起始页，简要介绍该主题的内容。每个主题之下再使用标题和小标题对所有图示进行细分，以便读者在目录中查找。

Structure

The book is divided into 14 major themes, each of which is preceded by a two-page spread with a short text introducing the context. Within each theme, titles and subtitles classify the illustrations into subcategories, which makes it easier to find them in the table of contents. The book also has a glossary of 45 common anatomical terms and an index containing all of the terms, titles, illustration titles and subtitles used in the book.

细胞结构

人体的所有细胞都有类似结构：最里面的是细胞核，细胞核的周围是细胞质。细胞的最外层是细胞膜，细胞膜包裹着整个细胞。

structure of a cell
All human cells have a similar structure: they are formed of a nucleus surrounded by cytoplasm and encased in a membrane.

细胞核

细胞的中央核心。以DNA的形式携带着遗传信息，并可调控蛋白质的合成。

cell nucleus
Central core of the cell containing genetic information in the form of DNA and guiding protein synthesis.

细胞质

液体物质。构成细胞的内部。包绕在细胞核的周围，其中散布着多种细胞器。

cytoplasm
Liquid substance forming the inside of the cell, around the nucleus, in which cellular organelles bathe.

高尔基体

细胞结构。由一组薄膜囊组成。参与细胞内蛋白质的加工完成和运输。

Golgi apparatus
Cell structure consisting of a group of membrane sacs; it is involved in the transport and maturation of proteins in the cell.

微丝

杆状结构。支撑细胞，细胞也因而得其形状。

microfilament
Rod-shaped structure supporting the cell and giving it its shape.

伪足

细胞质突起。属于某些特定细胞。主要在细胞位移时起作用。

pseudopod
Extension of the cytoplasm of certain cells, serving mainly in cell displacement.

微管

圆柱结构。支撑细胞，以便各种细胞器和物质在细胞内移动。

microtubule
Cylindrical structure supporting the cell and allowing organelles and substances in the cell to move about.

核糖体

细胞器。合成人体生长和功能所必需的多种蛋白质。游离在细胞质中或附着在内质网上。

ribosome
Organelle, floating free or bound to the endoplasmic reticulum, producing proteins essential to the formation and functioning of the human body.

线粒体

细胞结构。与细胞的呼吸活动相关，在细胞中生产和储存能量。

mitochondrion
Structure associated with cell breathing; it produces and stores energy in the cell.

液泡

泡状结构。储存水、代谢产物以及细胞所需的多种物质。

vacuole
Spherical cavity in which water, waste and various substances required by the cell are stored.

定义

定义对图示人体结构的本质特性、功能或特征给出说明。

DEFINITION
It explains the inherent qualities, function or characteristics of the element depicted in the illustration.

中心粒

细胞结构。在细胞进行有丝分裂时发挥关键作用。

centriole
Cell structure playing a key role during mitosis.

内质网

细胞结构。由膜管网组成。包裹细胞核，参与蛋白质合成。

endoplasmic reticulum
Cell structure consisting of a network of pockets surrounding the nucleus; it is involved in protein synthesis.

细胞膜

脂质双分子层。组成细胞的外表面。

cell membrane
Bilayer of lipid molecules forming the outer surface of the cell.

脂质

含有脂肪酸的分子。组成细胞膜。

lipids
Molecules containing fatty acids, making up the cell membrane.

蛋白质

有机化合物。由氨基酸组成。在细胞膜内形成通道，使细胞能与外部进行物质交换。

protein
Organic compound formed of amino acids; in the cell membrane, proteins form channels allowing the exchange of substances with the outside environment.

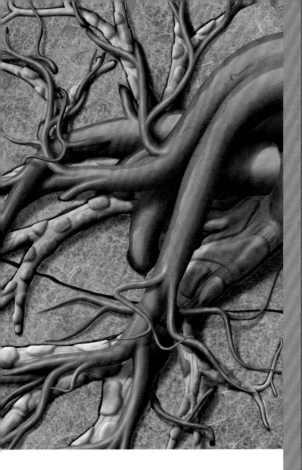

目录

目录

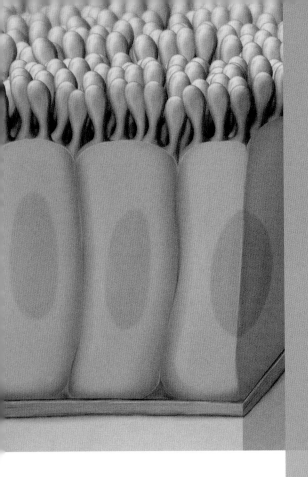

2
6
8
9

人体细胞 human cell

组织 tissue

有丝分裂 mitosis

脱氧核糖核酸 DNA

细胞与组织 Cell and tissues

人体的结构可分为几个层级，分别是组织、器官和系统。这些结构的基本单位都是细胞。细胞是生命活动的繁忙场所：细胞能集聚和传递能量、合成人体功能所必需的多种蛋白质，并能通过细胞分裂不断再生。细胞内也包含着我们每个人的全部基因。

The human body is formed of hierarchically organized components (tissues, organs, and systems), of which the basic unit is the cell. Cells are the site of intense activity: they accumulate and transmit energy, make proteins that are essential to the body's functioning, and constantly reproduce by cellular division. They also contain all of the genes belonging to each individual.

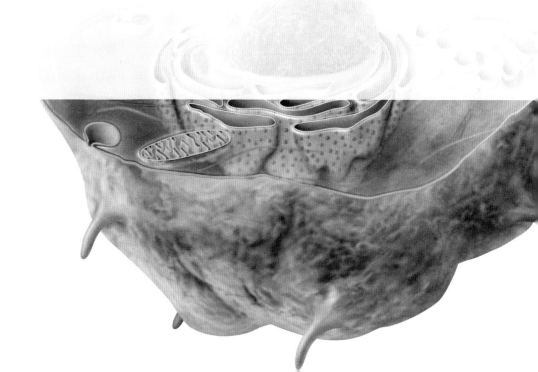

细胞结构
structure of a cell

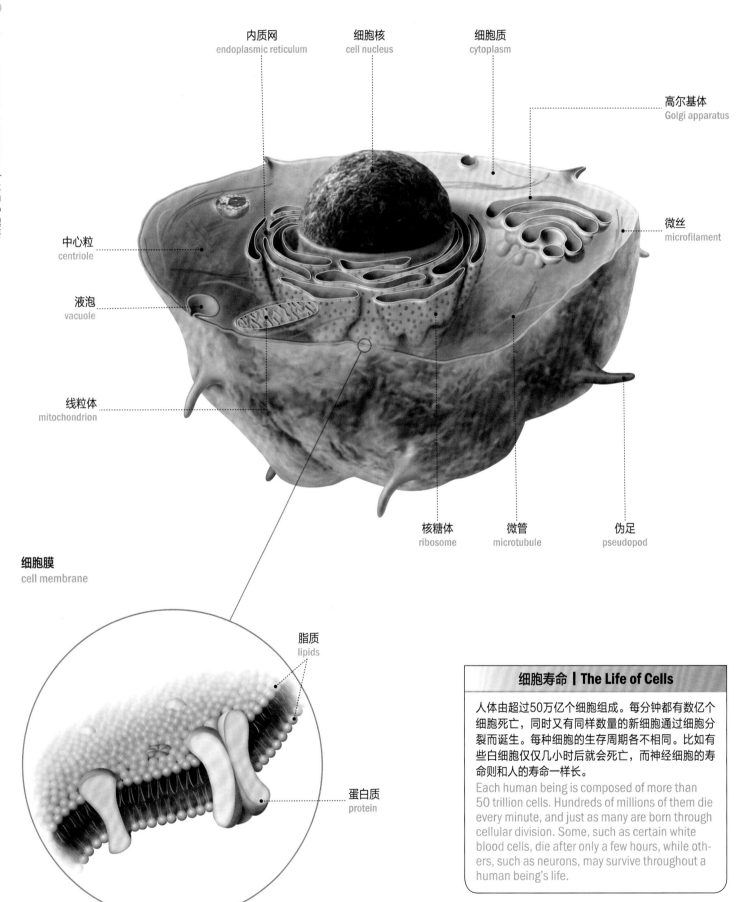

内质网
endoplasmic reticulum

细胞核
cell nucleus

细胞质
cytoplasm

高尔基体
Golgi apparatus

微丝
microfilament

中心粒
centriole

液泡
vacuole

线粒体
mitochondrion

核糖体
ribosome

微管
microtubule

伪足
pseudopod

细胞膜
cell membrane

脂质
lipids

蛋白质
protein

细胞寿命 | The Life of Cells

人体由超过50万亿个细胞组成。每分钟都有数亿个细胞死亡，同时又有同样数量的新细胞通过细胞分裂而诞生。每种细胞的生存周期各不相同。比如有些白细胞仅仅几小时后就会死亡，而神经细胞的寿命则和人的寿命一样长。

Each human being is composed of more than 50 trillion cells. Hundreds of millions of them die every minute, and just as many are born through cellular division. Some, such as certain white blood cells, die after only a few hours, while others, such as neurons, may survive throughout a human being's life.

细胞结构

人体的所有细胞都有类似结构：最里面的是细胞核，细胞核的周围是细胞质。细胞的最外层是细胞膜，细胞膜包裹着整个细胞。

structure of a cell
All human cells have a similar structure: they are formed of a nucleus surrounded by cytoplasm and encased in a membrane.

细胞核
细胞的中央核心。以DNA的形式携带着遗传信息，并可指导蛋白质的合成。

cell nucleus
Central core of the cell containing genetic information in the form of DNA and guiding protein synthesis.

细胞质
液体物质。构成细胞的内部。包绕在细胞核的周围，其中散布着多种细胞器。

cytoplasm
Liquid substance forming the inside of the cell, around the nucleus, in which cellular organelles bathe.

高尔基体
细胞结构。由一组薄膜囊组成。参与细胞内蛋白质的加工完成和运输。

Golgi apparatus
Cell structure consisting of a group of membrane sacs; it is involved in the transport and maturation of proteins in the cell.

微丝
杆状结构。支撑细胞，细胞也因而得其形状。

microfilament
Rod-shaped structure supporting the cell and giving it its shape.

伪足
细胞质突起。属于某些特定细胞。主要在细胞位移时起作用。

pseudopod
Extension of the cytoplasm of certain cells, serving mainly in cell displacement.

微管
圆柱结构。支撑细胞，以便各种细胞器和物质在细胞内移动。

microtubule
Cylindrical structure supporting the cell and allowing organelles and substances in the cell to move about.

核糖体
细胞器。合成人体生长和功能所必需的多种蛋白质。游离在细胞质中或附着在内质网上。

ribosome
Organelle, floating free or bound to the endoplasmic reticulum, producing proteins essential to the formation and functioning of the human body.

线粒体
细胞结构。与细胞的呼吸活动相关，在细胞中生产和储存能量。

mitochondrion
Structure associated with cell breathing; it produces and stores energy in the cell.

液泡
泡状结构。储存水、代谢产物以及细胞所需的多种物质。

vacuole
Spherical cavity in which water, waste and various substances required by the cell are stored.

中心粒
细胞结构。在细胞进行有丝分裂时发挥关键作用。

centriole
Cell structure playing a key role during mitosis.

内质网
细胞结构。由膜管网组成。包裹细胞核，参与蛋白质合成。

endoplasmic reticulum
Cell structure consisting of a network of pockets surrounding the nucleus; it is involved in protein synthesis.

细胞膜

脂质双分子层。组成细胞的外表面。

cell membrane
Bilayer of lipid molecules forming the outer surface of the cell.

脂质
含有脂肪酸的分子。组成细胞膜。

lipids
Molecules containing fatty acids, making up the cell membrane.

蛋白质
有机化合物。由氨基酸组成。在细胞膜内形成通道，使细胞能与外部进行物质交换。

protein
Organic compound formed of amino acids; in the cell membrane, proteins form channels allowing the exchange of substances with the outside environment.

细胞核
cell nucleus

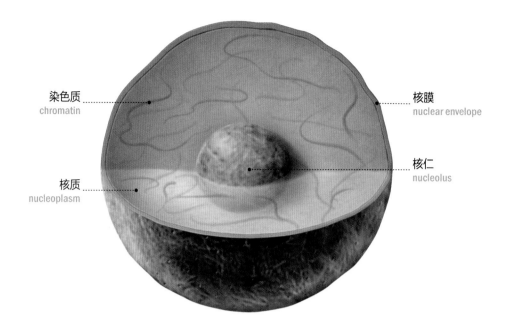

染色质
chromatin

核膜
nuclear envelope

核仁
nucleolus

核质
nucleoplasm

细胞举例
examples of cells

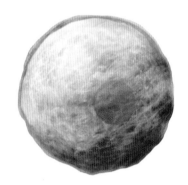

卵子
ovum

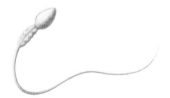

精子
spermatozoon

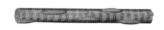

肌纤维
muscle fiber

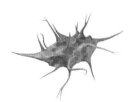

骨细胞
osteocyte

软骨细胞
chondrocyte

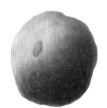

脂肪细胞
fat cell

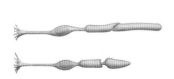

感光细胞
photoreceptor cell

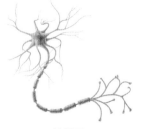

神经元
neuron

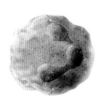

白细胞
white blood cell

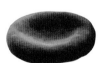

红细胞
red blood cell

细胞核

细胞的中央核心。以DNA的形式携带遗传信息，调控蛋白质的合成。

cell nucleus
Central core of the cell containing genetic information in the form of DNA and guiding protein synthesis.

染色质

由蛋白质和DNA组成的物质。位于细胞核中。在有丝分裂时，聚缩成染色体。

chromatin
Substance consisting of proteins and DNA contained in the nucleus; it is compressed into chromosomes during mitosis.

核膜

薄膜。包裹着细胞核。

nuclear envelope
Membrane surrounding the nucleus.

核质

液体物质。构成细胞核的内部。染色质与核仁散布于其中。

nucleoplasm
Liquid substance forming the inside of the nucleus of a cell and in which especially chromatin and nucleoli bathe.

核仁

位于细胞核内的球状体。参与核糖体的合成。

nucleolus
Spherical body located inside the nucleus and playing a role in the synthesis of ribosomes.

细胞举例

人体细胞大约有200种类型。取决于其在人体中所发挥的功能不同，不同种类细胞的形态和特性也都迥异。

examples of cells
The human body has about 200 types of cells, having very different characteristics and appearance depending on the functions that they perform in the organism.

卵子

成熟的女性生殖细胞。由卵巢产生。受精后，可使胚胎发育。

ovum
Mature female reproductive cell produced by the ovary; after fertilization by a spermatozoon, it enables an embryo to develop.

精子

成熟且具活力的男性生殖细胞。由睾丸产生，是精液的主要组成成分，其主要作用就是使卵子受精。

spermatozoon
Mature and mobile male reproductive cell produced by the testis; the main constituent of sperm, its purpose is to fertilize the ovum.

肌纤维

可收缩的细胞，是肌肉的组成成分。

muscle fiber
Contractile cell, constituent element of muscles.

骨细胞

成熟细胞。骨组织的组成成分。

osteocyte
Mature cell, constituent element of bone tissue.

软骨细胞

细胞。软骨的组成成分。

chondrocyte
Cell, constituent element of cartilage.

脂肪细胞

细胞。组成脂肪组织的主要成分。确保脂肪的合成、储存和释放。

fat cell
Cell forming the essential component of adipose tissue and ensuring the synthesis, storage and release of lipids.

感光细胞

视网膜上的细胞。能够捕捉光线并将其转换成神经信号。

photoreceptor cell
Cell found in the retina capable of capturing light rays and translating them into nerve signals.

神经元

神经系统细胞。使信息能以电信号和化学信号的形式进行传递。

neuron
Cell of the nervous system allowing information to be carried in the form of electrical and chemical signals.

白细胞

血液细胞。属于免疫系统，在人体防御中起关键的作用。

white blood cell
Blood cell belonging to the immune system, thus playing an essential role in the body's defenses.

红细胞

血液细胞。将氧气从肺输送到身体各组织，并将二氧化碳从身体各组织送回到肺。

red blood cell
Blood cell that carries oxygen from the lungs to the tissues and carbon dioxide from the tissues to the lungs.

组织

结构相似并发挥相似作用或互补作用的一类细胞。构成人体器官的细胞主要有以下四种：上皮细胞、结缔细胞、肌肉细胞和神经细胞。

tissue

All the cells that have a similar structure and perform similar or complementary functions. Four main cell types make up the frame of the organism: epithelial, connective, muscle and nervous.

上皮

组织。由分层排列的细胞组成。具有覆盖、分泌和保护的功能。

epithelium

Tissue formed of cells organized in layers; it serves covering, secretory and protective functions.

上皮细胞
组成上皮组织的细胞。

epithelial cell
Cell component of epithelial tissue.

微绒毛
细胞膜的表面突起。可增大细胞膜的表面。

microvillus
Protrusion of the cell membrane that increases its surface.

基膜
细胞外基质。可将上皮细胞固定到毗邻组织。

basal lamina
Extracellular matrix anchoring epithelial cells to adjacent tissue.

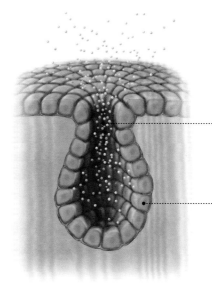

上皮组织举例

上皮组织包括：被覆上皮组织［外覆于整个体表和内衬于各腔体（黏膜、内皮、表皮）］和腺上皮组织（具有分泌功能）。

examples of epithelia

They include tissues that form the covering of all body surfaces and line inner cavities (mucous membranes, endothelia, epidermis), and glandular tissues that have secretory functions.

外分泌腺

将分泌细胞产生的分泌物排出体外的腺体。唾液腺和汗腺就是这类腺体。

exocrine gland

All secretory cells producing secretions released outside the body; they consist especially of salivary and sweat glands.

分泌导管
导管。可传送外分泌腺的分泌物。

excretory duct
Duct carrying secretions from the exocrine gland.

分泌细胞
上皮细胞。负责分泌人体所需的各种物质。

secretory cell
Epithelial cell specialized in the secretion of various substances useful to the body.

黏膜

湿润的上皮组织。内衬于人体的敞口腔体。在吸收和分泌（黏液）中发挥作用。

mucous membrane

Damp epithelial tissue lining an open cavity of the body; the mucous membrane plays a role in absorption and secretion (mucus).

黏液
半透明的黏性物质。由黏膜分泌，具有保护作用。

mucus
Translucent viscous substance secreted by the mucous membrane and that plays a protective role.

黏液细胞
上皮细胞。可分泌黏液。

mucous cell
Epithelial cell that secretes mucus.

上皮组织
由分层排列的细胞组成。具有覆盖、分泌和保护的功能。

epithelium
Tissue formed of cells organized in layers; it serves covering, secretory and protective functions.

黏液腺
外分泌腺。主要作用是分泌黏液。

mucous gland
Exocrine gland that secretes mainly mucus.

绒毛膜
疏松结缔组织。位于黏膜上皮组织的下方。

chorion
Loose connective tissue beneath the epithelial tissue of the mucous membrane.

黏膜肌层
一层薄薄的平滑肌组织。位于绒毛膜下方。

muscularis mucosae
Fine layer of smooth tissue beneath the chorion.

黏膜下层
结缔组织。位于黏膜下方。

submucosa
Connective tissue beneath the mucous membrane.

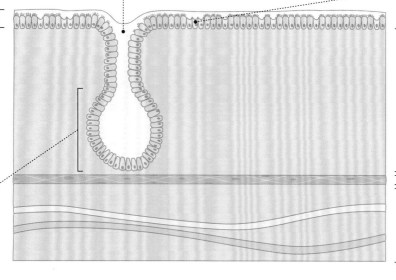

结缔组织举例

结缔组织：由相对较少的细胞和纤维散布于相对较多的细胞间质中组成。其功能包括支持、保护和填充间隙。

examples of connective tissues
Connective tissue: tissue made up of relatively few cells and fibers bathed in a more or less abundant fluid; its functions are to support, protect and fill in spaces.

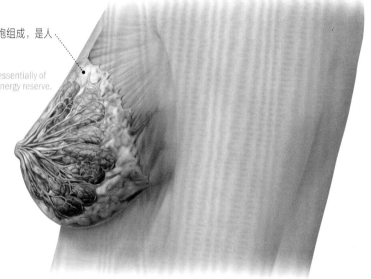

纤维组织

结缔组织。以富含胶原纤维为特征，主要用以形成肌腱和韧带。

fibrous tissue
Connective tissue characterized by an abundance of collagen fibers; it forms especially the tendons and ligaments.

脂肪组织

结缔组织。主要由脂肪细胞组成，是人体能量的储藏所在。

adipose tissue
Connective tissue made up essentially of adipocytes; it is the body's energy reserve.

软骨

结缔组织。由坚韧的细胞间质包裹软骨细胞形成。除了覆盖在骨关节面，还组成人体的某些柔软部位。

cartilage
Connective tissue consisting of cells encased in a rigid substance; it covers the articular surfaces of bones and forms certain soft parts of the body.

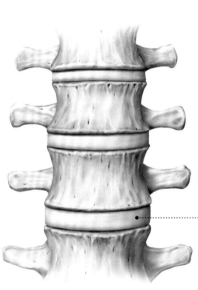

弹性组织

结缔组织。主要由弹性纤维组成。主要见于某些韧带以及动脉血管壁、气管壁和声带壁。

elastic tissue
Connective tissue made up predominantly of elastic fibers; it is found especially in certain ligaments and in the walls of the arteries, trachea and vocal chords.

最多见的组织 | The Most Abundant

结缔组织是人体中最多见的组织，存在于所有器官，占全部组织总体积的2/3。
Connective tissue, present in all organs, is the most abundant tissue in the human body: it accounts for two thirds of the total volume of tissue.

有丝分裂 | mitosis

有丝分裂
细胞分裂的一种机制。由一个母细胞形成
完全相同的两个子细胞。

mitosis
All the mechanisms of cell division that allow
the formation of two identical daughter cells
from a mother cell.

分裂前期
有丝分裂的第一阶段。在该阶段染色质浓缩成为
染色体。两对中心粒分别向相反的两极移动。

prophase
First stage of mitosis, during which the chromatin condenses into chromosomes; the two
pairs of centrioles move toward opposite poles.

分裂中期
有丝分裂的第二阶段。在纺锤体的引导下，
染色体在细胞中间排成一行，核膜破裂。

metaphase
Second stage of mitosis, during which the
chromosomes align in the middle of the
cell, guided by the mitotic spindle; the
nuclear membrane disaggregates.

分裂间期
两次细胞分裂之间的间隔时期。细胞
在此期间生长。

interphase
Period between two successive cell
divisions, during which the cell grows.

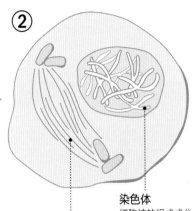

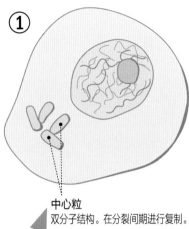

染色体
细胞核的组成成分。由DNA和多种
蛋白质组成，携带遗传信息。染色
体仅在细胞分裂的过程中出现。

chromosomes
Elements of the nucleus of a cell,
made up of DNA and proteins and
carrying genetic information; they are
observed only during cell division.

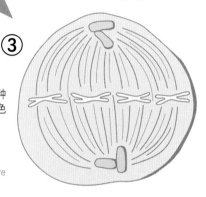

中心粒
双分子结构。在分裂间期进行复制。

centrioles
Double cellular structures that dupli-
cate during interphase.

有丝分裂纺锤体
短时间存在的细胞结构。在有丝分裂
时连接两对中心粒。

mitotic spindle
Ephemeral cellular structure joining the
two pairs of centrioles during mitosis.

分裂后期
有丝分裂的第三阶段。染色体分裂成染
色单体并向细胞的两极移动。

anaphase
Third stage of mitosis, during which the
chromosomes separate into chromatids
and move to either of the cell's poles.

胞质分裂
有丝分裂的一个阶段。细胞质一分为二，初始细
胞（母细胞）被两个完全相同的子细胞取代。

cytokinesis
Stage of mitosis during which the cytoplasm
separates in two; the original cell (or mother
cell) is replaced by two identical daughter cells.

分裂末期
有丝分裂的第四阶段。染色体又变回染色
质。新的核膜出现并分隔包裹两个细胞核。

telophase
Fourth stage of mitosis, during which the
chromosomes reassume the appearance
of the chromatin; a new nuclear envelope
appears to cordon off the two nuclei.

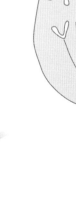

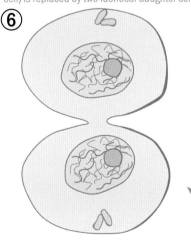

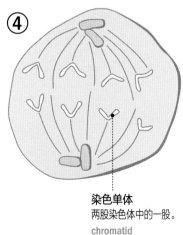

染色单体
两股染色体中的一股。

chromatid
One of the two strands of
a chromosome.

细胞质
凝胶样物质。组成细胞的内部，包
绕在细胞核周围。

cytoplasm
Gel-like substance forming the inside
of the cell, around the cell nucleus.

亿万个拷贝 ｜ Billions of Copies

人的遗传物质包含在46条染色体内（22对常染色体和1对性染色体）。人体每个细胞都有这些染色体的拷贝。例如，皮肤细胞也含有眼睛颜色的遗传指令。

The human genetic heritage is included in 46_chromosomes (22 pairs of autosomes and 1_pair of sex chromosomes). Each cell in the body has its own copy: for example, a skin cell contains the instruction for eye color.

脱氧核糖核酸分子
DNA分子呈双螺旋结构，由数十亿个核苷酸组成，是人体内的最大分子。

DNA molecule
The DNA molecule appears in the shape of a double helix made up of billions of nucleotides; it is the largest molecule in the human body.

脱氧核糖核酸
复杂大分子。DNA内携带每个人的遗传信息（基因）。

DNA
Complex molecule containing the genetic characteristics (genes) of every person.

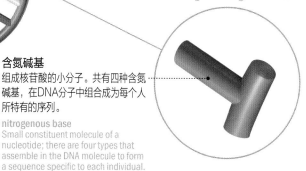

腺嘌呤
与胸腺嘧啶互补的含氮碱基。

adenine
Complementary nitrogenous base of thymine.

胸腺嘧啶
与腺嘌呤互补的含氮碱基。

thymine
Complementary nitrogenous base of adenine.

核苷酸
组成DNA分子的基本单位。核苷酸带有一个含氮碱基。

nucleotide
Basic unit of DNA molecules, consisting of a nitrogenous base.

胞嘧啶
与鸟嘌呤互补的含氮碱基。

cytosine
Complementary nitrogenous base of guanine.

鸟嘌呤
与胞嘧啶互补的含氮碱基。

guanine
Complementary nitrogenous base of cytosine.

含氮碱基
组成核苷酸的小分子。共有四种含氮碱基，在DNA分子中组合成为每个人所特有的序列。

nitrogenous base
Small constituent molecule of a nucleotide; there are four types that assemble in the DNA molecule to form a sequence specific to each individual.

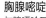

常染色体
染色体。携带与性别无关的遗传信息。

autosome
Chromosome that carries hereditary characteristics unrelated to sex.

性染色体
决定性别的染色体。

sex chromosomes
Chromosomes responsible for determining sex.

染色体
细胞核的组成成分。由DNA和多种蛋白质组成，携带遗传信息，仅在细胞分裂的过程中出现。

chromosomes
Elements of the nucleus of a cell, made up of DNA and proteins and carrying genetic information; they are observed only during cell division.

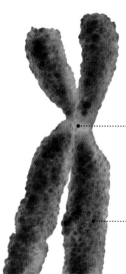

着丝点
短点。将两条染色单体连接在一起。

centromere
Short section of a chromosome that holds the two chromatids together.

染色单体
两股染色体中的一股。每条单体都有一支短臂和一支长臂。细胞分裂时，两条染色单体在着丝点分离。

chromatid
One of two strands of a chromosome, consisting of a short arm and a long arm; during cell division, the two chromatids separate at the centromere.

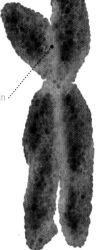

X染色体
性染色体。男女共有。

X chromosome
Sex chromosome present in both men and women.

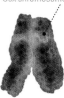

Y染色体
性染色体。仅男性有。

Y chromosome
Sex chromosome present only in men.

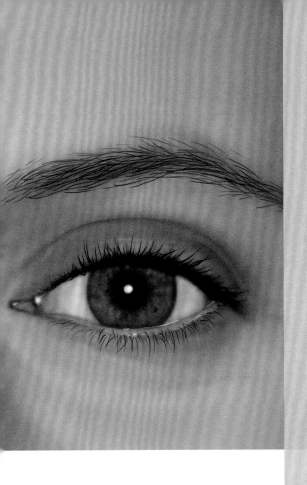

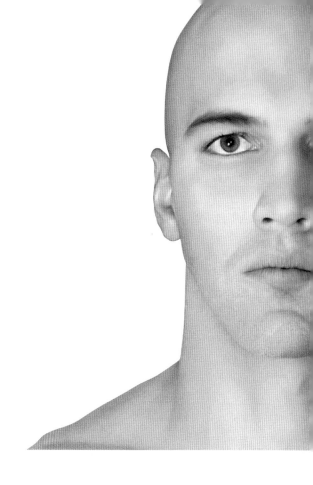

人体形态 Morphology

人体主要分为四个解剖部分：头部包含主要的感觉器官；躯干包含大部分内脏器官；上肢提供抓握能力；下肢使人能够移动和站立。这些部分通过多种多样的关节相互连接，使人体各部既能做出各种独立动作，也能做出复杂的联合动作。

The human body is divided into four main anatomical regions: the head, which contains the main sensory organs; the trunk, which contains most of the internal organs; the upper limbs, which provide gripping ability; and the lower limbs, which allow for locomotion and an upright posture. These parts are linked to each other by complex joints, which enable them to make independent and very complex movements.

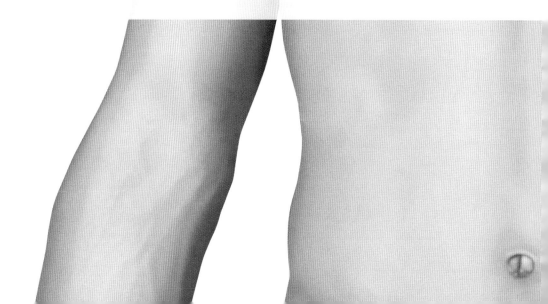

男人 | man

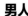

男人

具有男性性别的人类。男人的骨骼一般比女人的
更大更重。男人能够生成精子，使卵子受精。

man

Human being of the male sex whose skeleton is
generally larger and heavier than that of the female; he produces cells able to fertilize the ovum.

男人前面观
man: anterior view

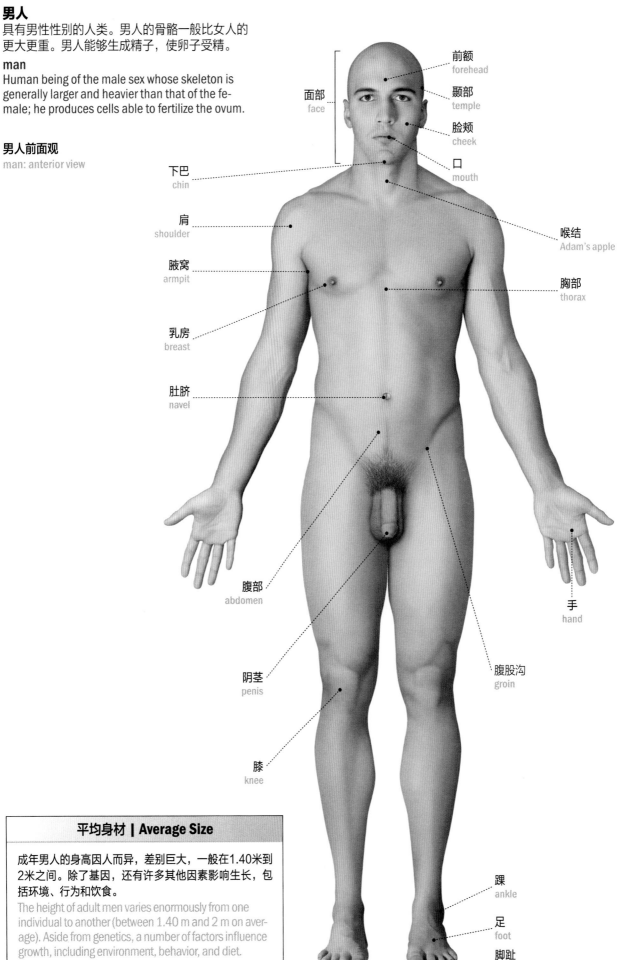

面部
face

前额
forehead

颞部
temple

脸颊
cheek

口
mouth

下巴
chin

肩
shoulder

腋窝
armpit

乳房
breast

肚脐
navel

喉结
Adam's apple

胸部
thorax

手
hand

腹部
abdomen

阴茎
penis

膝
knee

腹股沟
groin

踝
ankle

足
foot

脚趾
toe

平均身材 | **Average Size**

成年男人的身高因人而异，差别巨大，一般在1.40米到
2米之间。除了基因，还有许多其他因素影响生长，包
括环境、行为和饮食。

The height of adult men varies enormously from one
individual to another (between 1.40 m and 2 m on average). Aside from genetics, a number of factors influence
growth, including environment, behavior, and diet.

人体形态 | MORPHOLOGY

面部
头的前部。
face
Front part of the head.

下巴
面部下面的突出部分。与下颌骨相连。
chin
Protruding part of the lower face, corresponding to the mandible.

肩
关节。连接上臂和胸部。
shoulder
Joint connecting the arm with the thorax.

腋窝
在上臂和胸部之间的凹隙。位于肩关节下方。青春期始被覆毛发。
armpit
Hollow located beneath the shoulder between the arm and thorax and covered with hair at puberty.

乳房
前胸部包含乳头的部分。对于男性来说，乳房几乎没有发育，也没有什么特别的作用。
breast
Front part of the thorax containing the nipple; in men, the breast is barely developed and plays no particular role.

肚脐
圆形凹陷疤痕。由脐带切断后所形成。
navel
Scar in the form of a rounded depression resulting from the cutting of the umbilical cord.

腹部
躯干的下部分。位于横膈膜下方。其内主要包含消化系统、泌尿系统和生殖系统的相关器官。
abdomen
Lower part of the trunk, beneath the diaphragm, containing the main organs of the digestive, urinary and reproductive systems.

阴茎
可勃起的男性器官。用于性交和排尿。
penis
Erectile organ of men allowing copulation and voiding of urine.

膝
关节。连接大腿和小腿。
knee
Joint connecting the thigh with the leg.

前额
面部的上面。位于眉毛、发际线和颞部之间。
forehead
Upper part of the face between the eyebrows, hairline and temples.

颞部
头部的侧面。位于前额、眼睛、脸颊和耳朵之间。
temple
Side of the head between the forehead, eye, cheek and ear.

脸颊
面部的侧面。包含有能做出许多不同表情的肌肉。
cheek
Side of the face containing muscles capable of giving it many different expressions.

口
消化道的起始段。由嘴唇包围的一个空腔（口腔）组成。可以消化食物，并具有味觉、语言和呼吸的功能。
mouth
Initial part of the digestive tube made up of a cavity (oral cavity) surrounded by lips; it allows the ingestion of food and plays a role in tasting, speaking and breathing.

喉结
男人脖子上的突出部分。由喉部的两条软骨汇接而成。
Adam's apple
Protrusion of men's necks, formed by the joining of two strips of cartilage from the larynx.

胸部
躯干的上部分。位于横膈膜上方，其内主要包含心脏和肺。
thorax
Upper part of the trunk, above the diaphragm, containing especially the heart and lungs.

手
上肢的末端。具有触觉和抓握功能。
hand
Terminal part of the upper limb having a tactile and prehensile function

腹股沟
腹部和大腿交界处的凹陷。
groin
Depression located at the junction of the abdomen and thigh.

踝
关节。连接足和小腿。
ankle
Joint connecting the foot with the leg.

足
下肢的末端。人体直立时，足部支撑地面。
foot
Terminal part of the lower limb, resting on the ground during upright stance.

脚趾
足的延伸。由几个关节连接的骨（趾骨）组成，其末端有指甲覆盖。
toe
Extension of the foot, made up of several articulated bones (phalanges) and whose terminal end is covered with a nail.

男人后面观
man: posterior view

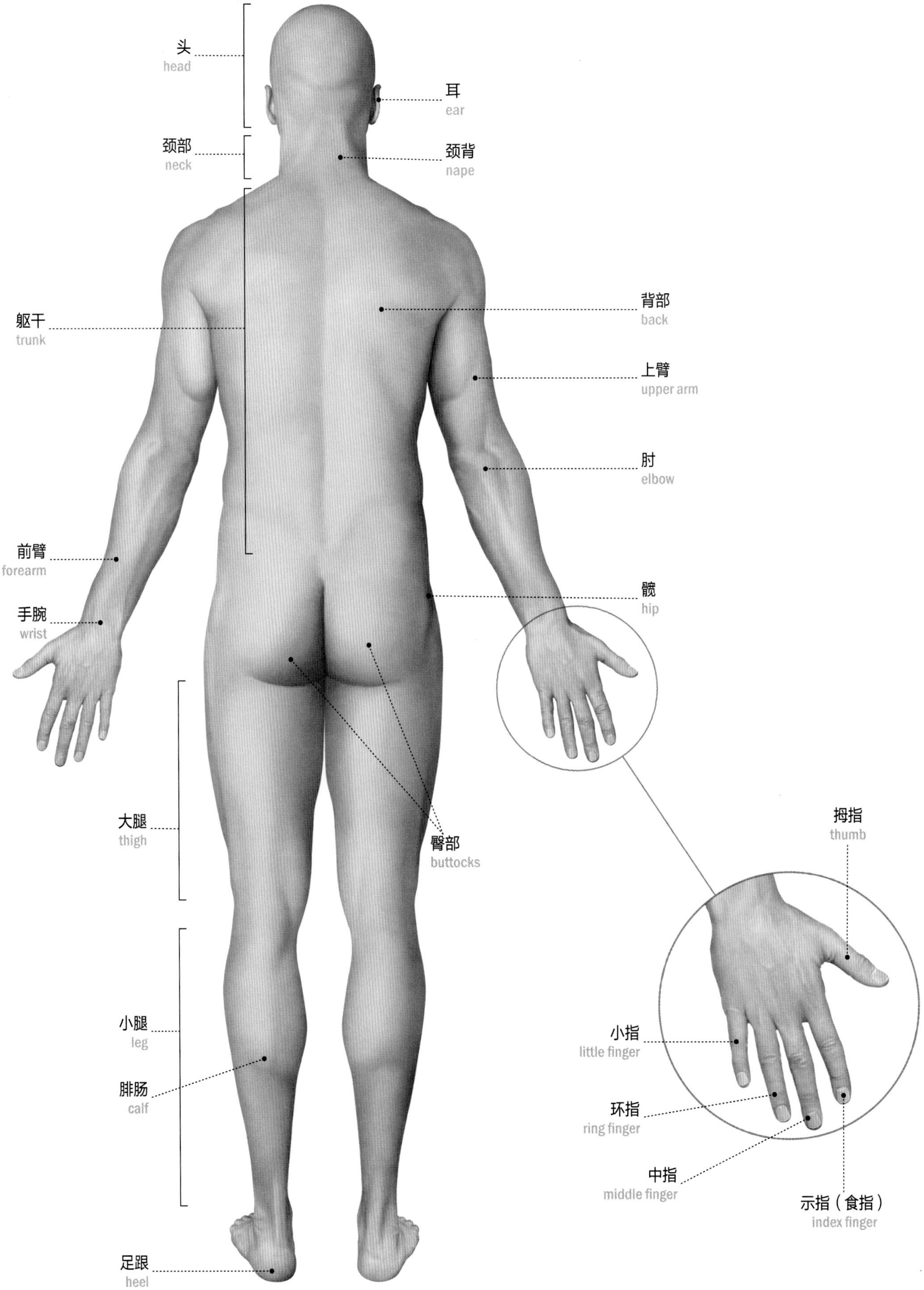

头
head

耳
ear

颈部
neck

颈背
nape

躯干
trunk

背部
back

上臂
upper arm

肘
elbow

前臂
forearm

髋
hip

手腕
wrist

拇指
thumb

大腿
thigh

臀部
buttocks

小指
little finger

环指
ring finger

小腿
leg

腓肠
calf

中指
middle finger

示指（食指）
index finger

足跟
heel

头
身体的最上部。靠颈部支撑，包含大脑和主要的感觉器官。
head
Upper part of the body, supported by the neck and containing the main sensory organs and brain.

颈部
连接头部和躯干，包含颈椎和喉部。
neck
Part of the body joining the head to the trunk and containing especially the cervical vertebrae and larynx.

躯干
由胸部和腹部组成，躯干上连接着头部和四肢。
trunk
Part of the body formed by the thorax and abdomen, to which the head and limbs are attached.

前臂
从肘到腕的上肢部分。
forearm
Part of the upper limb between the elbow and wrist.

手腕
关节。连接手与前臂。
wrist
Joint connecting the hand with the forearm.

大腿
从臀到膝的下肢部分。对应着股骨。
thigh
Part of the lower limb between the hip and knee, corresponding to the femur.

小腿
从膝到踝的下肢部分。
leg
Part of the lower limb between the leg and ankle.

腓肠
小腿后部。由小腿三头肌组成。
calf
Hind part of the leg, made up of triceps surae.

足跟
足的后部。对应跟骨。
heel
Hind part of the foot, corresponding to the calcaneus.

耳
听觉和平衡器官。由三部分组成：外耳、中耳和内耳。
ear
Organ of hearing and balance made up of three parts: the outer ear, the middle ear and the inner ear.

颈背
颈的后部。主要由肌肉构成。
nape
Hind part of the neck made up mainly of muscles.

背部
胸部的后侧。
back
Hind part of the thorax.

上臂
从肩到肘的上肢部分。对应着肱骨。
upper arm
Part of the upper limb between the shoulder and elbow, corresponding to the humerus.

肘
关节。连接上臂与前臂，由肱骨下端、桡骨上端和尺骨上端组成。
elbow
Joint between the arm and forearm, formed by the lower extremity of the humerus and the upper extremities of the radius and ulna.

髋
关节。连接下肢与骨盆。
hip
Joint connecting the leg with the pelvis.

臀部
丰满的部位。位于腰部下方，主要由肌肉组成。
buttocks
Fleshy parts located beneath the lumbar region, made up mainly of muscles.

拇指
第一根手指。短而有力，可与其余手指相对，便于抓握。
thumb
First digit of the hand, short and strong, opposable to the other digits to enable grasping.

示指（食指）
第二根手指。因常用来指向某处而得名。
index finger
Second digit of the hand, often used to point, hence its name

中指
第三根手指。也是最长的手指。
middle finger
Third and longest digit of the hand.

环指
第四根手指。因戒指通常戴在这根手指上而得名。
ring finger
Fourth digit of the hand; rings are traditionally worn on this finger, hence its name.

小指
第五根手指。也是最小的手指。
little finger
Fifth and smallest digit of the hand.

女人

具有女性性别的人类。能通过受精
卵怀孕。

woman

Human being of the female sex capable of conceiving children from an
ovum fertilized by a spermatozoon.

女人前面观
woman: anterior view

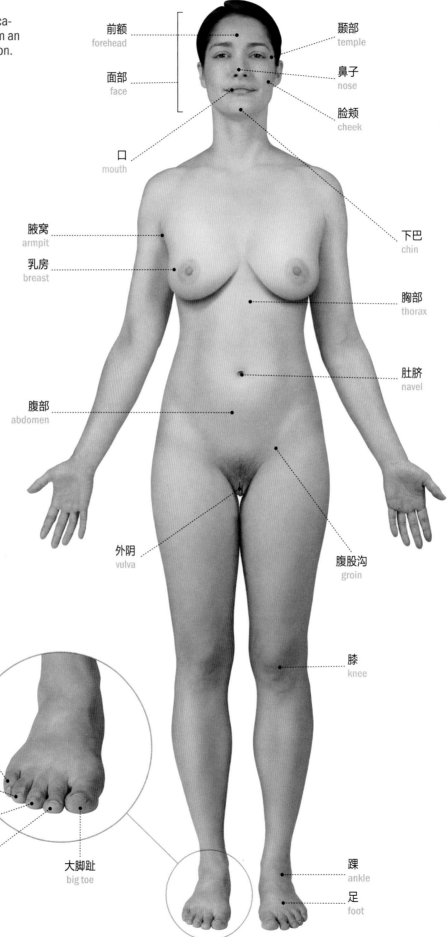

前额
forehead

面部
face

口
mouth

颞部
temple

鼻子
nose

脸颊
cheek

下巴
chin

腋窝
armpit

乳房
breast

胸部
thorax

肚脐
navel

腹部
abdomen

外阴
vulva

腹股沟
groin

膝
knee

小脚趾
little toe

第四脚趾
fourth toe

第三脚趾
third toe

第二脚趾
second toe

大脚趾
big toe

踝
ankle

足
foot

前额
面部的上部。位于眉毛、发际线和颞部之间。
forehead
Upper part of the face between the eyebrows, hairline and temples.

面部
头的前面。
face
Front part of the head.

口
消化道的起始段。由嘴唇包围的一个空腔（口腔）组成。可以消化食物，并具有味觉、语言和呼吸的功能。
mouth
Initial part of the digestive tube made up of a cavity (oral cavity) surrounded by lips; it allows the ingestion of food and plays a role in tasting, speaking and breathing.

腋窝
在上臂和胸部之间的凹隙。位于肩关节下方。青春期始被覆毛发。
armpit
Hollow located beneath the shoulder between the arm and thorax and covered with hair at puberty.

乳房
腺体器官。富含脂肪组织。包围胸肌并可分泌乳汁，哺乳新生儿。
breast
Glandular organ rich in adipose tissue, enclosing the pectoral muscles and secreting milk to feed the newborn after birth.

腹部
躯干的下部。位于横膈膜下方。其内主要包括消化系统、泌尿系统和生殖系统的相关器官。
abdomen
Lower part of the trunk, beneath the diaphragm, containing the main organs of the digestive, urinary and reproductive systems.

外阴
女性的所有外部生殖器官。可保护阴蒂和阴道口。
vulva
All the external female genital organs protecting the clitoris and vaginal opening.

小脚趾
最后一根足趾。也是最小的足趾。
little toe
Last and smallest toe of the foot.

第四脚趾
位于第三足趾和小趾之间。
fourth toe
Toe located between the third toe and little toe.

第三脚趾
位于第二足趾和第四足趾之间。
third toe
Toe located between the second toe and fourth toe.

第二脚趾
位于大脚趾和第三根足趾之间。
second toe
Toe located between the big toe and third toe.

大脚趾
第一根足趾。也是最大的足趾。
big toe
First and largest toe of the foot.

颞部
头的侧面。位于前额、眼睛、脸颊和耳朵之间。
temple
Side of the head between the forehead, eye, cheek and ear.

鼻子
面部中间的突出部分。有两个开孔（鼻孔），有嗅觉和呼吸功能。
nose
Protrusion in midsection of the face, with two orifices (nostrils), having an olfactory and respiratory function.

脸颊
面部的侧面。包含多个肌肉，可做出许多不同表情。
cheek
Side of the face containing muscles capable of giving it many different expressions.

下巴
面部下部的突出部分。与下颌骨相连。
chin
Protruding part of the lower face, corresponding to the mandible.

胸部
躯干的上部。位于横膈膜上方。其内主要包含心脏和肺。
thorax
Upper part of the trunk, above the diaphragm, containing especially the heart and lungs.

肚脐
圆形凹陷疤痕。由脐带切断后所形成。
navel
Scar in the form of a rounded depression resulting from the cutting of the umbilical cord.

腹股沟
位于下腹部和大腿的交界处的凹陷。
groin
Depression located at the junction of the abdomen and thigh.

膝
关节。连接大腿和小腿。
knee
Joint connecting the thigh with the leg.

踝
关节。连接足部和小腿。
ankle
Joint connecting the foot with the leg.

足
下肢的末端。人体直立时，足部支撑地面。
foot
Terminal part of the lower limb, resting on the ground during upright stance.

人体形态 | MORPHOLOGY

女人后面观
woman: posterior view

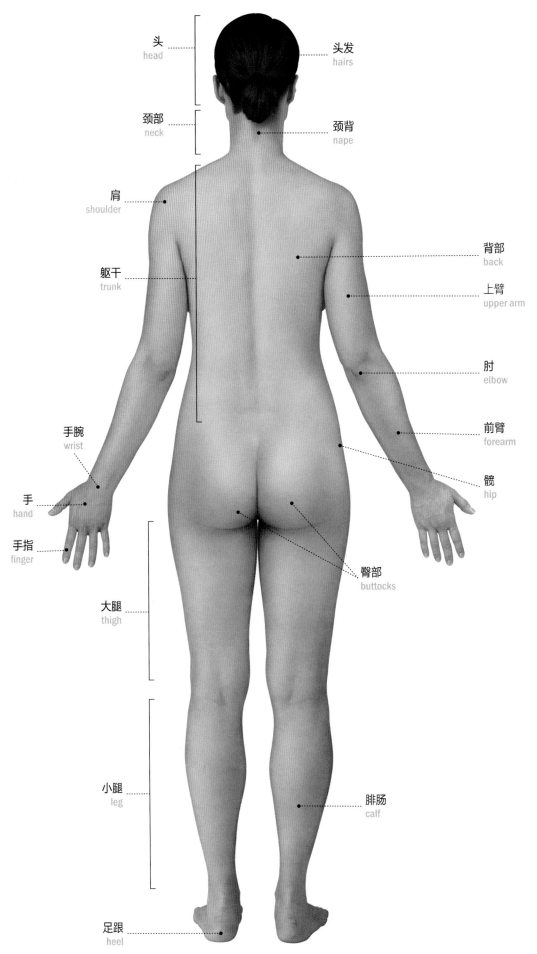

头
head

头发
hairs

颈部
neck

颈背
nape

肩
shoulder

背部
back

躯干
trunk

上臂
upper arm

肘
elbow

手腕
wrist

前臂
forearm

手
hand

髋
hip

手指
finger

臀部
buttocks

大腿
thigh

小腿
leg

腓肠
calf

足跟
heel

头
身体上部。由颈部支撑，包含主要感觉器官和大脑。
head
Upper part of the body, supported by the neck and containing the main sensory organs and brain.

颈部
连接头部和躯干，包含颈椎和喉部。
neck
Part of the body joining the head to the trunk and containing especially the cervical vertebrae and larynx.

肩
关节。连接手臂和胸部。
shoulder
Joint connecting the arm with the thorax.

躯干
由胸部和腹部组成，头部和四肢都连接于躯干。
trunk
Part of the body formed by the thorax and abdomen, to which the head and limbs are attached.

手腕
关节。连接手和前臂。
wrist
Joint connecting the hand with the forearm.

手
上肢的末端。具有触觉和抓握功能。
hand
Terminal part of the upper limb having a tactile and prehensile function.

手指
手的延伸。由各种关节连接的骨（指骨）组成，其末端有指甲覆盖。
finger
Extension of the hand, made up of various articulated bones (phalanges) and whose terminal end is covered with a nail.

大腿
从髋到膝的下肢部位。对应股骨。
thigh
Part of the lower limb between the hip and knee, corresponding to the femur.

小腿
从膝到踝的下肢部位。
leg
Part of the lower limb between the leg and ankle.

足跟
足的后部。对应跟骨。
heel
Hind part of the foot, corresponding to the calcaneus.

头发
覆盖头部的毛发。可保护颅部的皮肤，每个人头发的外形和颜色都不一样。
hairs
Filaments covering the head and protecting especially the skin of the skull; their appearance and color vary depending on the individual.

颈背
颈的后部。主要由肌肉组成。
nape
Hind part of the neck made up mainly of muscles.

背部
胸部的后面
back
Hind part of the thorax.

上臂
从肩到肘的上肢部分。对应着肱骨。
upper arm
Part of the upper limb between the shoulder and elbow, corresponding to the humerus.

肘
关节。连接上臂与前臂，由肱骨下端、桡骨上端和尺骨上端组成。
elbow
Joint between the arm and forearm, formed by the lower extremity of the humerus and the upper extremities of the radius and ulna.

前臂
从肘到腕的上肢部分。
forearm
Part of the upper limb between the elbow and wrist.

髋
关节。连接下肢和骨盆。
hip
Joint connecting the leg with the pelvis.

臀部
丰满的部位。位于腰部下方，主要由肌肉组成。
buttocks
Fleshy parts located beneath the lumbar region, made up mainly of muscles.

腓肠
小腿后部。由小腿三头肌构成。
calf
Hind part of the leg, made up of triceps surae.

水，生命之源 | Water: The Source of Life

女人身体的平均含水量为60%。人体含水量主要会因年龄不同而不同，但男人比女人的含水量要略高一些，这是因为男人的脂肪组织要比女人的少一些。
A woman's body contains an average of 60% water. This proportion, which varies mainly as a function of age, is slightly higher among men, who generally have a lower proportion of fat tissue.

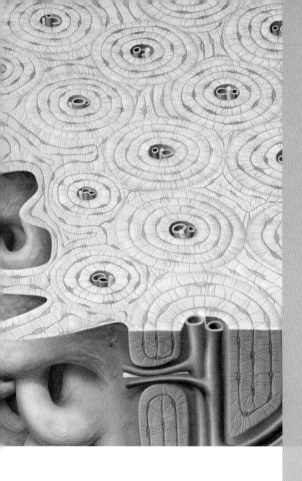

骨架 Skeleton

骨架是身体里所有骨骼的统称。骨骼通过关节相互连接。中轴骨架包括面颅骨、脑颅骨和脊柱，脊柱连接着肋骨。中轴骨架通过肩胛带与上肢相连，通过骨盆带与下肢相连。骨骼的每个部分都有其特定功能。中轴骨的骨骼支撑着身体，保护着重要器官，而四肢的骨骼则可以进行各种各样的运动，有助于身体稳定、行走和抓握。

The skeleton is all of the bones in the body, connected to each other by joints. The axial skeleton includes the bones of the face, the cranium, and the vertebral column, into which the ribs are inserted. It is connected to the upper limbs by the pectoral girdle and to the lower limbs by the pelvic girdle. Each part of the skeleton fulfills a specific function: the bones of the axial skeleton support the body and protect the vital organs, while the bones in the limbs allow a great variety of movements and contribute to the stability of the body, to walking, and to gripping ability.

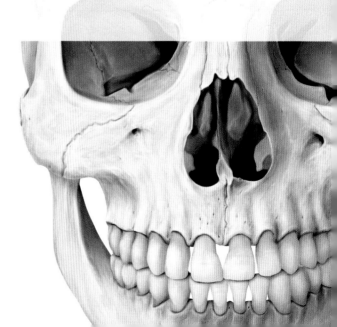

骨骼

坚硬结构，构成骨架。骨骼由关节相连，主要由富含矿物质的骨组织组成。

bones

Rigid structures making up the skeleton; connected by joints, they are largely made up of bone tissue rich in mineral salts.

骨骼类型

根据形状不同，将骨骼分为四种：扁骨、短骨、长骨和不规则骨。

types of bones

There are four bone types, classified according to their shape: flat, short, long and irregular.

长骨

长形管状骨。大小差别很大，主要组成上肢和下肢。

long bone

Elongated bone, varying greatly in size, making up especially the upper and lower limbs.

骨骺

长骨的末端。圆形。表面覆盖着关节软骨。

epiphysis

End of a long bone, rounded in shape and covered with articulating cartilage.

干骺端

长骨的一部分。位于骨干和骨骺之间。在骨的生长中起重要作用。

metaphysis

Part of a long bone between the diaphysis and epiphysis, playing an important role in the bone's growth.

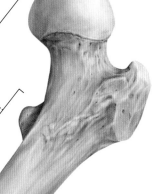

骨干

长骨的中间部分。呈圆柱形。

diaphysis

Middle part of a long bone, having a cylindrical shape.

扁骨

薄片状骨。在血细胞的生产中起重要作用。肩胛骨就是典型的扁骨。

flat bone

Thin, flat bone playing an important role in the production of blood cells; the shoulder blade is a typical example.

干骺端

长骨的一部分。位于骨干和骨骺之间。在骨的生长中起重要作用。

metaphysis

Part of a long bone between the diaphysis and epiphysis, playing an important role in the bone's growth.

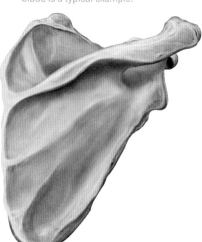

骨骺

长骨的末端。圆形，表面覆盖着关节软骨。

epiphysis

End of a long bone, rounded in shape and covered with articulating cartilage.

短骨

小块骨。呈大致的立方形。见于某些关节（踝部、腕部）。

short bone

Small bone, more or less cubic, found in some joints (ankles, wrists).

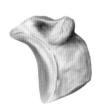

不规则骨

大小不同且形状复杂的骨头（如椎骨）。

irregular bone

Bone of varying size and complex shape (e.g., vertebrae).

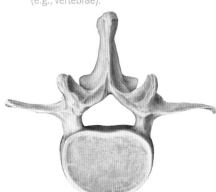

骨骼的强度大于钢 | Stronger than Steel

骨骼是人体内仅次于牙釉质的最坚硬的物质。其强度是同等重量钢的三倍。

After tooth enamel, bone is the hardest substance in the human body. A bone is three times stronger than a bar of steel of equal weight.

骨组织
坚实的结缔组织，富含钙和胶原蛋白，是骨骼的主要组成部分。
bone tissue
Solid connective tissue, rich in calcium and collagen, making up the major part of bones.

骨细胞
成熟细胞。骨骼组织的组成成分。
osteocyte
Mature cell, constituent element of bone tissue.

骨膜
纤维膜。覆盖骨骼。
periosteum
Fibrous membrane covering the bone.

骨单位
骨密质的基本组成单位。由胶原蛋白、血管、神经纤维和骨细胞组成。
osteon
Basic unit of compact bone tissue, made up of collagen, blood vessels, nerve fibers and osteocytes.

长骨横截面
cross section of a long bone

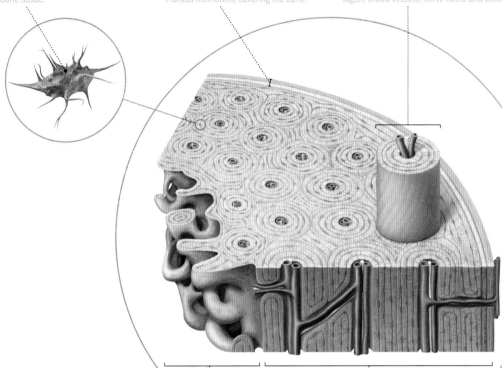

骨松质
构成骨骼内部的组织。由骨小梁组成，血管、神经纤维和红骨髓在骨小梁之间走行。
spongy bone tissue
Tissue forming the inner part of the bone, consisting of bony cords between which blood vessels, nerve fibers and red bone marrow are lodged.

骨密质
致密组织。能抵抗压力和冲击，构成骨骼的中间部分。
compact bone tissue
Dense tissue, resistant to pressure and shocks, forming the middle part of the bone.

股骨纵切面
longitudinal section of an adult femur

黄骨髓
富含脂质的软组织。位于成人长骨的髓腔内。
yellow bone marrow
Soft tissue, rich in lipids, located in the medullary cavity of long bones in adults.

骨密质
致密组织。能抵抗压力和冲击，构成骨骼的中间部分。
compact bone tissue
Dense tissue, resistant to pressure and shocks, forming the middle part of the bone.

髓腔
圆柱形空腔。位于长骨骨干的内核。成人的髓腔内含有黄骨髓。
medullary cavity
Cylindrical cavity in the inner core of the diaphysis of long bones, containing yellow bone marrow in adults.

骨松质
构成骨骼中间部分的组织。由骨小梁组成，血管、神经纤维和红骨髓在骨小梁之间走行。
spongy bone tissue
Tissue forming the inner part of the bone, consisting of bony cords between which blood vessels, nerve fibers and red bone marrow are lodged.

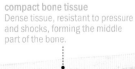

主要骨骼

人体骨架由206块大小不同、形状各异并以关节互连的骨骼组成。

main bones

The human skeleton is made up of 206 articulated bones of varying sizes and shapes.

骨架前面观

skeleton: anterior view

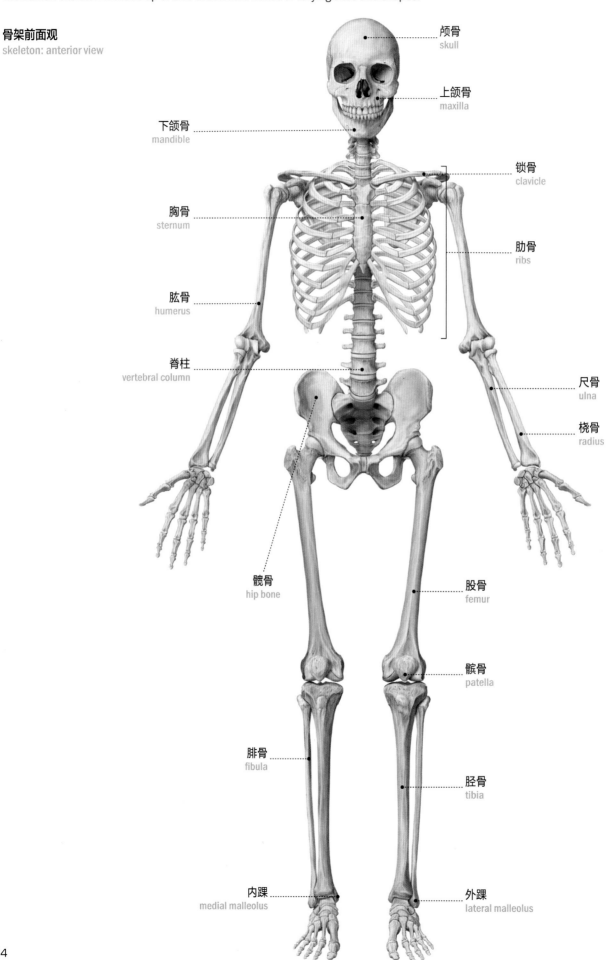

颅骨
skull

上颌骨
maxilla

下颌骨
mandible

锁骨
clavicle

胸骨
sternum

肋骨
ribs

肱骨
humerus

脊柱
vertebral column

尺骨
ulna

桡骨
radius

髋骨
hip bone

股骨
femur

髌骨
patella

腓骨
fibula

胫骨
tibia

内踝
medial malleolus

外踝
lateral malleolus

下颌骨

不成对的骨。组成下颚。与颞骨形成关节，以便咀嚼。

mandible
Unpaired bone forming the lower jaw, articulating with the temporal bones to allow chewing.

胸骨

垂直向下延伸的骨骼。形成胸廓的前中部，与肋软骨相连。

sternum
Vertically extended bone forming the anterior midsection of the thoracic cage and articulating with the costal cartilages.

肱骨

大型成对的骨。组成上臂骨架，在肩关节和肘关节之间。

humerus
Very large paired bone making up the skeleton of the arm, between the shoulder and elbow joints.

脊柱

由33块椎骨组成，从颅骨延伸到骨盆。支撑头部和躯干，内含脊髓。

vertebral column
Bony grouping of 33_vertebrae, extending from the skull to the pelvis; it supports the head and trunk and contains the spinal cord.

髋骨

成对的骨。组成骨盆的绝大部分，由3块在儿童时期不同的骨头融合而成：髂骨、耻骨和坐骨。

hip bone
Paired bone forming the largest part of the pelvis; it results from the fusion of three distinct bones in childhood; the ilium, the pubis and the ischium.

译者注：这3块骨在儿童期借软骨联合在一起，到成年后，3块骨在髋臼处愈合。

腓骨

成对的骨。组成小腿骨架外侧部分，在膝关节和踝关节之间。

fibula
Paired bone forming the outer part of the skeleton of the leg, between the knee and ankle joints.

内踝

内踝的骨性突起。由胫骨的骨骺形成。

medial malleolus
Bony protrusion of the inner ankle, formed by the epiphysis of the tibia.

颅骨

由八块骨（四块扁骨和四块不规则骨）组成的骨骼结构。覆盖并保护着脑。

skull
Bony structure formed of eight bones (four even bones and four odd bones) covering and protecting the brain.

上颌骨

成对的骨。组成上颚、部分硬腭、眼眶和鼻腔。

maxilla
Paired bone forming the upper jaw, part of the hard palate, orbits and nasal cavity.

锁骨

成对的骨。连接肩胛骨和胸骨。

clavicle
Paired bone connecting the shoulder blade to the sternum.

肋骨

12对呈弧形弯曲的骨。形成胸廓的外侧部分。

ribs
Bones (12_pairs) curved in the shape of an arc, forming the lateral parts of the thoracic cage.

尺骨

成对的骨。组成前臂骨架内侧部分，在肘关节和腕关节之间。

ulna
Paired bone forming the inner part of the skeleton of the forearm, between the elbow and wrist joints.

桡骨

成对的骨。组成前臂骨架外侧部分，在肘关节和腕关节之间。

radius
Paired bone forming the outer part of the skeleton of the forearm, between the elbow and wrist joints.

股骨

成对的骨。组成大腿的骨架，在髋关节和膝关节之间。

femur
Paired bone forming the skeleton of the thigh, between the hip and knee joints.

髌骨

成对的三角形骨。与股骨在膝部构成关节。

patella
Paired bone, triangular in shape, articulated with the femur at the knee.

胫骨

大型成对的骨。组成小腿骨骼的内侧部分。在膝关节和踝关节之间。

tibia
Very large paired bone forming the inner part of the skeleton of the leg, between the knee and ankle joints.

外踝

外踝的骨性突起。由腓骨的骨骺形成。

lateral malleolus
Bony protrusion of the outer ankle, formed by the epiphysis of the fibula.

骨架后面观
skeleton: posterior view

肩峰
acromion

肩胛骨
scapula

内上髁
medial epicondyle

外上髁
lateral epicondyle

鹰嘴
olecranon

髂骨
ilium

骶骨
sacrum

大转子
greater trochanter

耻骨
pubis

坐骨
ischium

尾骨
coccyx

股骨内侧髁
medial condyle of femur

股骨外侧髁
lateral condyle of femur

距骨
talus

跟骨
calcaneus

骨骼的大小 | The Size of Bones

人体有各种大小的骨骼。最长和最重的是股骨，仅股骨的长度就占了人体身高的1/4。股骨支撑着身体一半的重量。最小的骨是位于内耳的镫骨，长度仅为4毫米。

The human body contains bones in a wide variety of sizes. The longest and heaviest is the femur, which, alone, is one quarter the height of an individual and supports half of his weight. The smallest is the stapes bone, situated in the inner ear, which is barely 4_mm_long.

肩峰
肩胛骨的突起。与锁骨以关节相连。
acromion
Bony protrusion of the shoulder blade, articulating with the clavicle.

肩胛骨
与锁骨和肱骨相关联的成对的三角形骨。它保护胸腔，并作为一些背部肌肉的起止点。
scapula
Paired bone, triangular in shape, articulating with the clavicle and humerus; it protects the thorax and serves as the insertion point for several back muscles.

内上髁
肱骨下端内侧的突起。手和手指的屈肌止点。
medial epicondyle
Inner protrusion of the lower extremity of the humerus, serving to attach various flexor muscles of the hand and fingers.

鹰嘴
尺骨近端。与肱骨远端以关节相连。形成肘部突起。
olecranon
Upper extremity of the ulna articulating with the humerus and forming the protrusion of the elbow.

外上髁
肱骨下端外侧的突起。手和手指的伸肌的止点。
lateral epicondyle
Outer protrusion of the lower extremity of the humerus, serving to attach various extensor muscles of the hand and fingers.

骶骨
三角形骨。由五块骶椎骨融合而成。
sacrum
Triangular bone resulting from the fusion of five sacral vertebrae.

髂骨
髋骨的上部。呈喇叭形。
ilium
Upper part of the hip bone, flared in shape.

耻骨
髋骨的前部。在耻骨联合处连接。
pubis
Front part of the iliac bone, articulated at the level of the pubic symphysis.

大转子
股骨上端的突起。大腿和臀部的几块肌肉附着其上。
greater trochanter
Protrusion of the upper extremity of the femur, where several muscles of the thigh and buttock insert themselves.

尾骨
小型三角骨。在成年初始由四块尾椎骨融合而成，构成脊柱的下末端。
coccyx
Small triangular bone formed by the fusion, at the start of adulthood, of the four coccygeal vertebrae, and making up the lower extremity of the vertebral column.

坐骨
髋骨下部。
ischium
Lower part of the iliac bone.

股骨内侧髁
股骨下端内侧的圆形隆起。与胫骨形成关节。
medial condyle of femur
Rounded protrusion of the inner part of the lower extremity of the femur, allowing articulation with the tibia.

股骨外侧髁
股骨下端外侧的圆形隆起。与胫骨形成关节。
lateral condyle of femur
Rounded protrusion of the outer part of the lower extremity of the femur, allowing articulation with the tibia.

距骨
成对的跗骨。位于跟骨上，与胫骨和腓骨相连。
talus
Paired bone of the tarsus resting on the calcaneus and articulating with the tibia and fibula.

跟骨
成对的跗骨。形成足跟并连接跟腱和一些小腿肌肉。
calcaneus
Paired bone of the tarsus forming the heel of the foot and serving to attach the Achilles tendon and several calf muscles.

颅骨

由八块骨（四块扁骨和四块不规则骨）组成的骨骼结构。覆盖并保护着脑。

skull

Bony structure formed of eight bones (four even bones and four odd bones) covering and protecting the brain.

颅骨侧面观
skull: lateral view

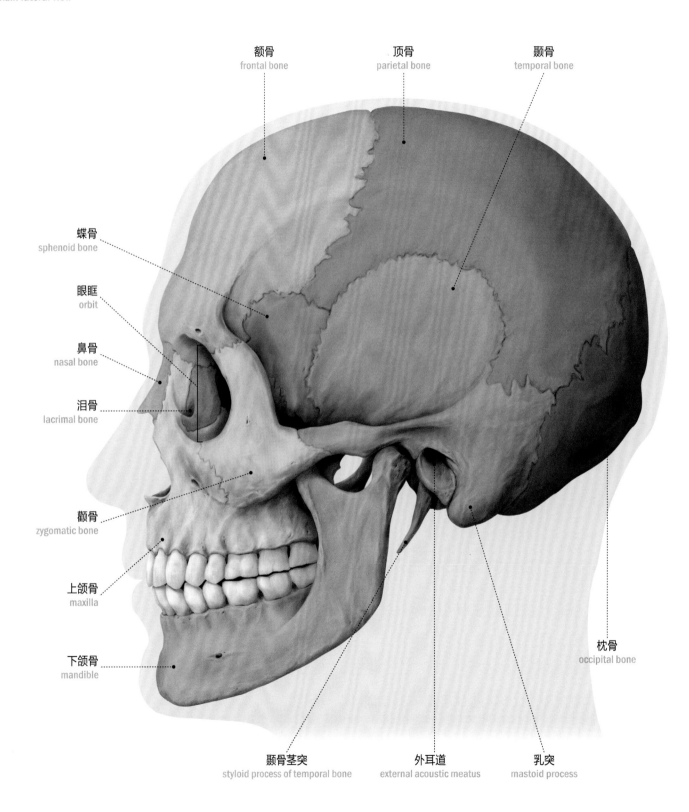

额骨
frontal bone

顶骨
parietal bone

颞骨
temporal bone

蝶骨
sphenoid bone

眼眶
orbit

鼻骨
nasal bone

泪骨
lacrimal bone

颧骨
zygomatic bone

上颌骨
maxilla

下颌骨
mandible

颞骨茎突
styloid process of temporal bone

外耳道
external acoustic meatus

乳突
mastoid process

枕骨
occipital bone

额骨
不成对的骨。构成颅骨前部（前额和眼眶顶部）。

frontal bone
Unpaired bone forming the front part of the skull (forehead and roof of the orbits).

蝶骨
不成对的骨。位于眼眶后方，与整个颅骨同宽。

sphenoid bone
Unpaired bone located behind the orbits and taking up the entire width of the skull.

眼眶
面部的两个骨性空腔。包含眼球、视神经和眼肌。

orbit
Each of two bony cavities of the face containing the eyeballs, optic nerves and ocular muscles.

鼻骨
面部中间两根相连的骨。构成鼻梁。

nasal bone
Each of two interarticulated bones in the middle of the face forming the bridge of the nose.

泪骨
成对的骨。构成部分眼眶的内侧壁。

lacrimal bone
Paired bone forming part of the medial wall of the orbit.

颧骨
成对的骨。构成颧骨以及眼眶的外侧壁。

zygomatic bone
Paired bone forming the cheekbone and lateral wall of the orbit.

上颌骨
成对的骨。构成上颌、部分硬腭、眼眶和鼻腔。

maxilla
Paired bone forming the upper jaw, part of the hard palate, orbits and nasal cavity.

下颌骨
不成对的骨。构成下颌，与颞骨形成关节，以便于咀嚼。

mandible
Unpaired bone forming the lower jaw, articulating with the temporal bones to allow chewing.

颞骨茎突
颞骨的骨性突出。又长又细，用于连接咽的韧带和肌肉。

styloid process of temporal bone
Bony protrusion of the temporal bone, long and slender, serving to attach ligaments and muscles of the pharynx.

顶骨
成对的骨。构成颅骨顶部的最大部分。

parietal bone
Paired bone making up the largest part of the roof of the skull.

颞骨
成对的骨。位于颅骨两侧，与下颌骨形成关节。

temporal bone
Paired bone located at the side of the skull, articulating with the mandible.

枕骨
不成对的骨。构成颅骨的后下部，保护小脑和脑干。

occipital bone
Unpaired bone forming the back and lower part of the skull, protecting the cerebellum and brain stem.

乳突
颞骨的骨性突起。有两个充满空气的空腔与中耳比邻。

mastoid process
Bony protrusion of the temporal bone, containing two air-filled cavities adjacent to the middle ear.

外耳道
骨性通道。耳廓收集到的声波由此到达鼓膜。

external acoustic meatus
Bony canal through which sounds captured by the pinna reach the eardrum.

骨架 | SKELETON

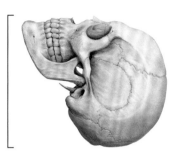

颅骨基底
bottom of skull

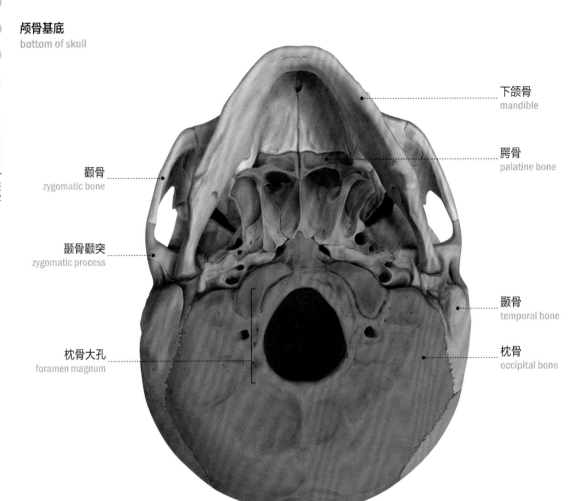

下颌骨
mandible

腭骨
palatine bone

颧骨
zygomatic bone

颞骨颧突
zygomatic process

枕骨大孔
foramen magnum

颞骨
temporal bone

枕骨
occipital bone

颅骨矢状面
sagittal section of skull

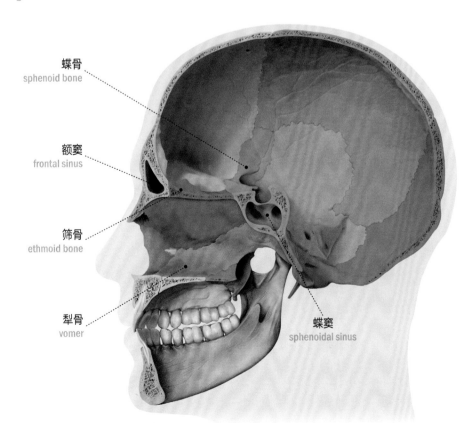

蝶骨
sphenoid bone

额窦
frontal sinus

筛骨
ethmoid bone

犁骨
vomer

蝶窦
sphenoidal sinus

可移动的骨 | Mobile Bones

人在出生时，组成颅骨的几块骨骼并非是完全融合在一起的。它们通过薄膜即囟门相连，因而具有一定的移动性。这使得新生儿的头部在分娩时能够发生形变。在出生后的最初几年里，也还能继续适应脑部的生长。

At birth, the bones of the skull are not totally fused. They are connected by membranes, the fontanels, and retain some mobility to enable the newborn's head to deform during birth, and then to allow the skull to adapt to the growth of the brain during the first years of life.

颧骨

成对的骨。构成颊骨及眼眶外侧壁。

zygomatic bone
Paired bone forming the cheekbone and lateral wall of the orbit.

下颌骨

不成对的骨。构成下颌，与颞骨形成关节，以便于咀嚼。

mandible
Unpaired bone forming the lower jaw, articulating with the temporal bones to allow chewing.

颞骨颧突

颞骨的突起。形成脸颊的上缘。

zygomatic process
Protrusion of the temporal bone, forming the upper limit of the cheek.

腭骨

不成对的骨。构成硬腭后部。

palatine bone
Unpaired bone forming the back of the hard palate.

颞骨

成对的骨。位于颅骨两侧，与下颌骨形成关节。

temporal bone
Paired bone located at the side of the skull, articulating with the mandible.

枕骨大孔

枕骨的孔。专供延髓通过。

foramen magnum
Aperture of the occipital bone through which the medulla oblongata especially passes.

枕骨

不成对的骨。构成颅骨的后下部，保护小脑和脑干。

occipital bone
Unpaired bone forming the back and lower part of the skull, protecting the cerebellum and brain stem.

蝶骨

不成对的骨。位于眼眶后方，与头颅同宽。

sphenoid bone
Unpaired bone located behind the orbits and taking up the entire width of the skull.

蝶窦

蝶骨的空腔。与鼻腔相通，加热吸入的空气。

sphenoidal sinus
Hollow cavity in the sphenoid bone, communicating with the nasal cavity and warming inhaled air.

额窦

额骨的空腔。与鼻腔相通，加热吸入的空气。

frontal sinus
Hollow cavity in the frontal bone, communicating with the nasal cavity and warming inhaled air.

筛骨

不规则不成对的骨。位于鼻腔后面，在面部和颅骨的结合部。

ethmoid bone
Irregular unpaired bone located behind the nasal cavity, at the juncture of the face and skull.

犁骨

成对的骨。位于鼻腔后部和下部。

vomer
Unpaired bone in the posterior and lower part of the nasal cavity.

脊柱 | vertebral column

脊柱
骨性轴体。由33块椎骨组成，从颅骨一直延伸到骨盆。脊柱支撑着头部和躯干，内含脊髓。

vertebral column
Bony axis consisting of 33 vertebrae extending from the skull to the pelvis; the vertebral column supports the head and trunk and contains the spinal cord.

枢椎
第二颈椎。上有垂直的突起，能使寰椎以其为轴，带动颅骨转动。

axis
Second cervical vertebra, having a vertical apophysis allowing the atlas to pivot and the skull to rotate.

隆椎
第7颈椎。有较长的棘突，是颈椎到胸椎的过渡。

vertebra prominens
Last cervical vertebra, having a protruding spiny apophysis and serving as a transition between the cervical and thoracic vertebrae.

椎间盘
圆形扁平软骨结构。分隔两块椎骨，具有弹性，赋予脊柱活动性。

intervertebral disk
Flat, rounded cartilaginous structure separating two vertebrae; its elasticity provides mobility to the vertebral column.

数量不等 | A Variable Number

形成尾骨的尾椎数目因人而异。大多数人有四块，但有些人有三块或五块。

The number of coccygeal vertebrae forming the coccyx may vary from individual to individual. Most people have four, but some have three or five.

骶骨
三角形骨。由5块骶椎骨融合而成。

sacrum
Triangular bone resulting from the fusion of five sacral vertebrae

尾骨
小三角形骨。在成年初期，4块尾骨融合成尾椎，构成脊柱的下末端。

coccyx
Small triangular bone formed by the fusion, at the start of adulthood, of the four coccygeal vertebrae, and making up the lower extremity of the vertebral column.

脊柱前面观
vertebral column: anterior view

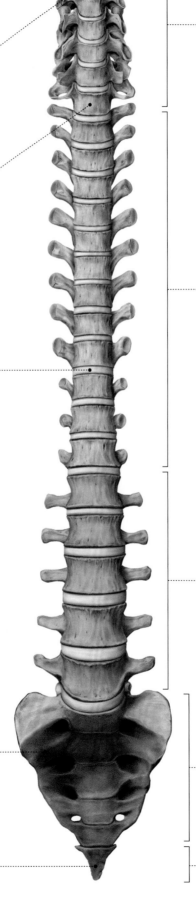

寰椎
第一颈椎，与颅骨在枕骨大孔处相连。

atlas
First cervical vertebra, articulating with the skull at the foramen magnum.

颈椎
非常灵活的椎骨，共7节。位于颈部，构成脊柱的上部分。

cervical vertebrae
Highly mobile vertebrae (7) forming the upper part of the vertebral column at the neck.

胸椎
椎骨（共12节），位于胸廓，支撑肋骨。

thoracic vertebrae
Vertebrae (12) supporting the ribs, located at the thorax.

腰椎
大块椎骨（共5节），胸椎下方，位于腹部。

lumbar vertebrae
Massive vertebrae (5) beneath the thoracic vertebrae at the abdomen.

骶椎
腰椎下方的5块椎骨融合而成骶骨。

sacral vertebrae
Vetebrae (5) beneath the lumbar vertebrae fusing to form the sacrum.

尾椎
骶骨下方的4块椎骨融合而成尾骨。

coccygeal vertebrae
Vertebrae (4) beneath the sacrum fusing to form the coccyx.

骨架 | SKELETON

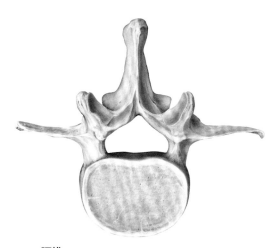

颈椎
高活动性的椎骨。共7节,位于颈部,构成脊柱的
上部分。

cervical vertebra
Each of seven highly mobile vertebrae forming the
upper part of the vertebral column at the neck.

脊柱侧面观
vertebral column: lateral view

颈椎前凸
脊柱在颈椎部位的正常凹形生理弯曲。

cervical lordosis
Normal concave curvature of the vertebral column at the cervical vertebrae.

胸椎后凸
脊柱在胸椎部位的正常凸形生理弯曲。

kyphosis
Normal convex curvature of the vertebral
column at the thoracic vertebrae.

腰椎前凸
脊柱在腰椎部位的正常的凹形生理弯曲。

lumbar lordosis
Normal concave curvature of the vertebral
column at the lumbar vertebrae.

腰椎
胸椎下方的大块椎骨。共5块,位于腹部。

lumbar vertebra
Each of five massive vertebrae located beneath
the thoracic vertebrae at the abdomen.

胸椎
支撑肋骨的椎骨。共12块,位于胸部。

thoracic vertebra
Each of 12 vertebrae supporting the
ribs, located at the thorax.

椎弓根
有多个突起的骨性结构。组成椎体后部。

vertebral arch
Bony element comprising the posterior part of a
vertebra and having several apophyses.

棘突
椎骨后部的骨性突起。用于连接背部肌肉和韧带。

spinous process
Bony protrusion behind a vertebra serving to attach
the muscles and ligaments of the back.

横突
椎体侧面的骨性突起。用于连接韧带。

transverse process
Bony protrusion on the side of a vertebra
serving to attach ligaments.

关节突
椎弓上的骨性突起,使相邻椎骨形成关节。

articular process
Bony outgrowth on the neural arch of a vertebra allowing it to articulate with adjacent
vertebrae.

椎孔
由椎体和椎弓组成的孔。用于容纳脊髓。

vertebral foramen
Aperture bordered by the vertebral body
and neural arch of a vertebra, housing the
spinal cord.

椎体
厚圆盘状骨。组成椎体前部。

vertebral body
Thick disk-shaped bony element comprising
the anterior part of a vertebra.

胸廓

骨性结构。由12对肋骨、12块胸椎以及胸骨组成。包围并保护胸腔的器官，在呼吸中发挥作用。

thoracic cage

Bony structure consisting of 12 pairs of ribs, 12 thoracic vertebrae and the sternum; it encloses and protects the organs of the thorax and plays a role in breathing.

胸廓前面观
thoracic cage: anterior view

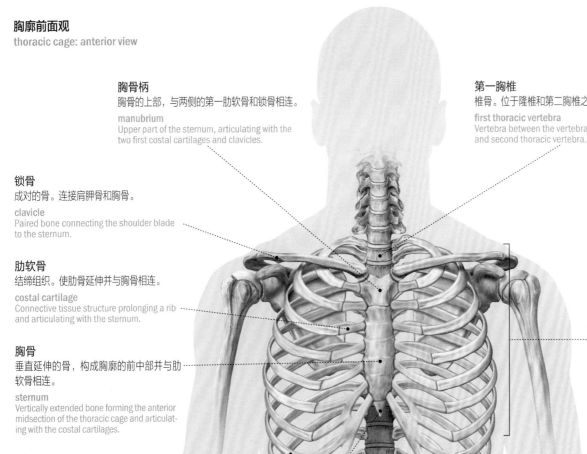

胸骨柄
胸骨的上部，与两侧的第一肋软骨和锁骨相连。
manubrium
Upper part of the sternum, articulating with the two first costal cartilages and clavicles.

第一胸椎
椎骨。位于隆椎和第二胸椎之间。
first thoracic vertebra
Vertebra between the vertebra prominens and second thoracic vertebra.

锁骨
成对的骨。连接肩胛骨和胸骨。
clavicle
Paired bone connecting the shoulder blade to the sternum.

肋软骨
结缔组织。使肋骨延伸并与胸骨相连。
costal cartilage
Connective tissue structure prolonging a rib and articulating with the sternum.

胸骨
垂直延伸的骨，构成胸廓的前中部并与肋软骨相连。
sternum
Vertically extended bone forming the anterior midsection of the thoracic cage and articulating with the costal cartilages.

真肋
胸廓上部的肋骨（7对）。各有各的肋软骨。
true ribs
Ribs (7 pairs) having their own costal cartilage, located in the upper part of the thoracic cage.

肋弓
真肋下方的肋骨（有3对）。共用肋软骨。
false ribs
Ribs (3 pairs) sharing the same costal cartilage, located beneath the true ribs.

浮肋
构成胸廓下部的肋骨（2对）。其前端不附着在胸骨上。
floating ribs
Ribs (2 pairs) whose anterior extremity is not attached to the sternum, forming the lower part of the thoracic cage.

剑突
胸骨下末端的三角形骨突。
xiphoid process
Triangular bony outgrowth at the lower extremity of the sternum.

第十二胸椎
最后一节胸椎。位于第十一胸椎和第一腰椎之间。
twelfth thoracic vertebra
Last thoracic vertebra between the eleventh thoracic vertebra and the first lumbar vertebra.

胸廓横切面
transverse section of thoracic cage

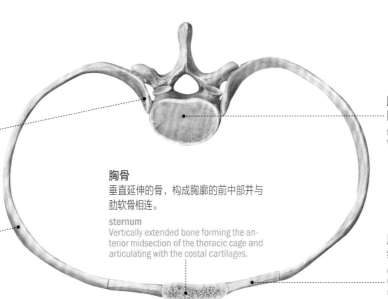

肋骨头
肋骨的后末端。通过两个接触点与胸椎相连。
head of rib
Posterior extremity of a rib, articulating with a thoracic vertebra via two contact points.

胸椎
胸部支撑肋骨的椎骨，共12块。
thoracic vertebra
Vertebra at the thorax, supporting the ribs.

肋骨
圆弧形骨。构成胸廓外部。
rib
Bone, curved in an arc, forming the lateral parts of the thoracic cage.

胸骨
垂直延伸的骨，构成胸廓的前中部并与肋软骨相连。
sternum
Vertically extended bone forming the anterior midsection of the thoracic cage and articulating with the costal cartilages.

肋软骨
结缔组织。使肋骨延伸并与胸骨相连。
costal cartilage
Connective tissue structure prolonging a rib and articulating with the sternum.

骨盆
环状骨带。由骶骨、尾骨和两个髂骨组成。连接下肢和中轴骨。

pelvis
Bony girdle consisting of the sacrum, coccyx and two iliac bones, joining the bones of the lower limbs to the axial skeleton.

男性骨盆前面观
man's pelvis: anterior view

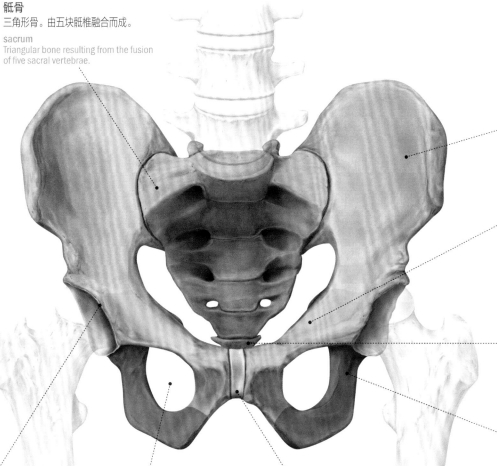

骶骨
三角形骨。由五块骶椎融合而成。

sacrum
Triangular bone resulting from the fusion of five sacral vertebrae.

髂骨
髂骨的上部，呈喇叭形。

ilium
Upper part of the iliac bone, flared in shape.

耻骨
髂骨的前部。在耻骨联合处连接。

pubis
Front part of the iliac bone, articulated at the level of the pubic symphysis.

尾骨
小三角形骨。在成年初期，四块尾骨融合成尾椎，构成脊柱的下末端。

coccyx
Small triangular bone formed by the fusion, at the start of adulthood, of the four coccygeal vertebrae, and making up the lower extremity of the vertebral column.

坐骨
髂骨的下部。

ischium
Lower part of the iliac bone.

髋臼
髂骨的凹腔处。股骨头在其中形成关节。

acetabulum
Cavity of the iliac bone within which the head of the femur articulates.

闭孔
髂骨上的孔。以耻骨、坐骨和髋臼为界。几乎完全被一层膜封闭。

obturator foramen
Aperture of the iliac bone bordered by the pubis, ischium and acetabulum; it is almost entirely enclosed in a membrane.

耻骨联合
几乎不活动的软骨关节。连接两块耻骨。

pubic symphysis
Cartilaginous joint with little mobility, connecting the two pubes

女性骨盆前面观
女人的骨盆比男人的更大、更浅，特征是坐骨的间隔更宽。

A woman's pelvis: anterior view
A woman's pelvis is larger and shallower than a man's and is characterized by more widely spaced ischia.

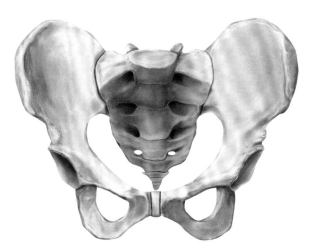

特有的步态 | A Typical Step

女性骨盆骨骼的特有排列方式改变了髋臼的方向，使女性在走路时呈现出特有的步态，臀部会左右摇摆。

The particular arrangement of bones in a woman's pelvis changes the orientation of the acetabulum, which causes the swaying hips typical of a woman's walk.

手 | hand

手

上肢的末端。具有触觉和抓握功能，手部骨架有27块骨。

hand

Terminal part of the upper limb, having a tactile and prehensile function. The skeleton of the hand has 27 bones.

手前面观
hand: anterior view

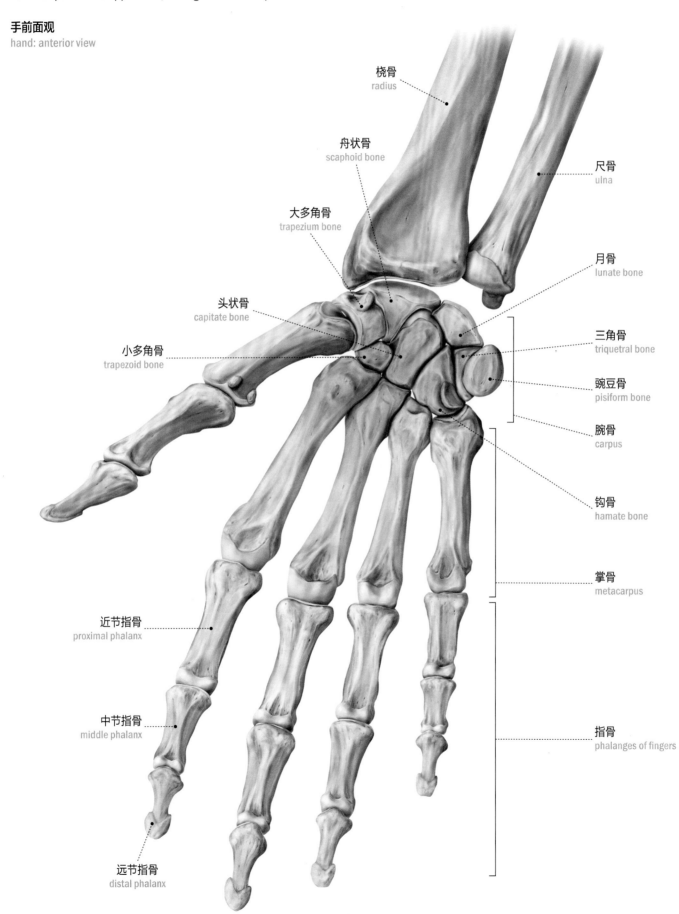

桡骨
radius

舟状骨
scaphoid bone

尺骨
ulna

大多角骨
trapezium bone

月骨
lunate bone

头状骨
capitate bone

三角骨
triquetral bone

小多角骨
trapezoid bone

豌豆骨
pisiform bone

腕骨
carpus

钩骨
hamate bone

掌骨
metacarpus

近节指骨
proximal phalanx

中节指骨
middle phalanx

指骨
phalanges of fingers

远节指骨
distal phalanx

桡骨
肘关节和腕关节之间的骨。构成前臂骨架外侧部分。

radius
Bone forming the outer part of the skeleton of the forearm, between the elbow and wrist joints.

尺骨
肘关节和腕关节之间的骨，构成前臂骨架内侧部分。

ulna
Bone forming the inner part of the skeleton of the forearm, between the elbow and wrist joints.

舟状骨
近排腕骨。在手腕处与桡骨相连。

scaphoid bone
Bone of the upper row of the carpus articulating with the radius at the wrist.

月骨
半月形近排腕骨。在手腕处与桡骨相连。

lunate bone
Semilunar bone of the upper row of the carpus articulating with the radius at the wrist.

大多角骨
远排腕骨。与第一掌骨相连。

trapezium bone
Bone of the lower row of the carpus articulating with the first metacarpal.

三角骨
近排腕骨。在手腕处与尺骨相连。

triquetral bone
Bone of the upper row of the carpus articulating with the ulna at the wrist.

头状骨
远排腕骨，与第三掌骨相连，腕骨中最大的一块。

capitate bone
Bone of the lower row of the carpus articulating with the third metacarpal; it is the largest of the carpal bones.

豌豆骨
近排腕骨。是腕骨中最小的骨。

pisiform bone
Bone of the upper row of the carpus; it is the smallest of the carpal bones.

小多角骨
远排腕骨。与第二掌骨相连。

trapezoid bone
Bone of the lower row of the carpus articulating with the second metacarpal.

腕骨
组成腕关节骨架的八块骨。

carpus
Group of eight bones (carpal bones) making up the skeleton of the wrist.

近节指骨
手指的第一指骨。与掌骨相连。

proximal phalanx
First phalanx of the finger, connected to the metacarpal.

钩骨
远排腕骨。与第四和第五掌骨相连。

hamate bone
Bone of the lower row of the carpus articulating with the fourth and fifth metacarpals.

中节指骨
手指的第二指骨。

middle phalanx
Second phalanx of the finger.

掌骨
构成手掌的五根骨。连接远排腕骨和近节指骨。

metacarpus
All five bones (metacarpals) forming the palm of the hand, connecting the upper row of the carpus with the proximal phalanges.

远节指骨
手指的第三指骨。

distal phalanx
Third phalanx of the finger.

指骨
构成手指的骨骼。除了拇指有两节指骨外，其余每个手指都有三节指骨。

phalanges of fingers
Bones forming the skeleton of the fingers. Each finger has three phalanges, except the thumb that has two.

足 | foot

足
下肢的末端。站立时支撑于地面，由26块骨组成。

foot
Terminal part of the lower limb, resting on the ground during upright stance; the skeleton of the foot has 26 bones.

足前面观
foot: anterior view

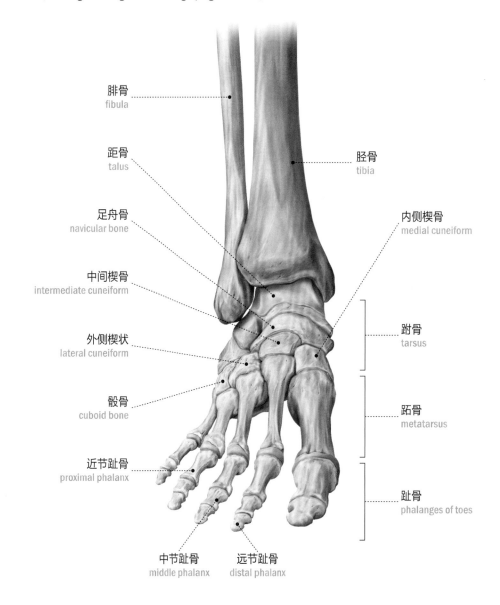

腓骨
fibula

距骨
talus

足舟骨
navicular bone

中间楔骨
intermediate cuneiform

外侧楔状
lateral cuneiform

骰骨
cuboid bone

近节趾骨
proximal phalanx

胫骨
tibia

内侧楔骨
medial cuneiform

跗骨
tarsus

跖骨
metatarsus

趾骨
phalanges of toes

中节趾骨
middle phalanx

远节趾骨
distal phalanx

足侧面观
foot: lateral view

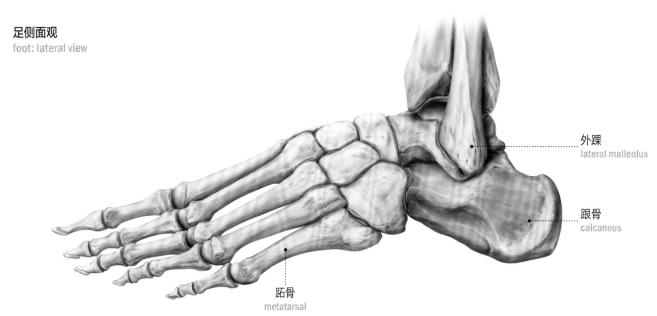

外踝
lateral malleolus

跟骨
calcaneus

跖骨
metatarsal

腓骨
在膝关节和踝关节之间，构成小腿骨架的外部。
fibula
Bone forming the outer part of the skeleton of the leg, between the knee and ankle joints.

距骨
位于跟骨上方，与胫骨和腓骨相连的跗骨。
talus
Bone of the tarsus resting on the calcaneus and articulating with the tibia and fibula.

足舟骨
跗骨中的一块。呈扁平状，与距骨和三块楔骨相连。
navicular bone
Flat bone of the tarsus articulating with the talus and the three cuneiform bones.

中间楔骨
与第二跖骨相连的跗骨。
intermediate cuneiform
Bone of the tarsus articulating with the second metatarsal.

外侧楔骨
与第三跖骨相连的跗骨。
lateral cuneiform
Bone of the tarsus articulating with the third metatarsal.

骰骨
与第四和第五跖骨相连的跗骨。
cuboid bone
Bone of the tarsus articulating with the fourth and fifth metatarsals.

近节趾骨
足趾的第一趾骨。与跖骨相连。
proximal phalanx
First phalanx of the toe, connected to the metatarsal.

外踝
外踝的骨性凸起。由腓骨的骨骺形成。
lateral malleolus
Bony protrusion of the outer ankle, formed by the epiphysis of the fibula.

跟骨
构成足跟，跟腱与小腿的若干肌肉附着的跗骨。
calcaneus
Bone of the tarsus forming the heel of the foot and serving to attach the Achilles tendon and several calf muscles.

胫骨
在膝关节和踝关节之间，形成小腿骨架内部的大型骨骼。
tibia
Very large bone forming the inner part of the skeleton of the leg, between the knee and ankle joints.

内侧楔骨
与第一跖骨相连的跗骨。
medial cuneiform
Bone of the tarsus articulating with the first metatarsal.

跗骨
组成踝关节骨架的七块骨（跗骨）。
tarsus
Group of seven bones (tarsal bones) forming the skeleton of the ankle.

跖骨
五块骨（跖骨）组成，构成脚掌，连接前排跗骨和近节趾骨。
metatarsus
Group of five bones (metatarsals) making up the sole of the foot and connecting the front row of the tarsus with the proximal phalanges of the toes.

趾骨
构成足趾骨架的骨。除了第一足趾有两块趾骨外，其余足趾都有三块趾骨。
phalanges of toes
Bones forming the skeleton of the toes. Each toe has three phalanges, except for the big toe that has two.

远节趾骨
足趾的第三趾骨。
distal phalanx
Third phalanx of the toe.

中节趾骨
足趾的第二趾骨。
middle phalanx
Second phalanx of the toe.

骨骼密集区 | Concentration of Bones

手和足总共有106块骨，超过人体骨骼总数的一半。
In total, the hands and feet contain 106 bones-more than half of all the bones in the human body.

跖骨
由足部的五块骨构成。
metatarsal
Each of five bones of the foot forming the metatarsus.

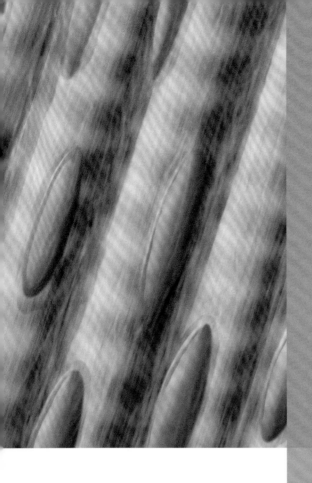

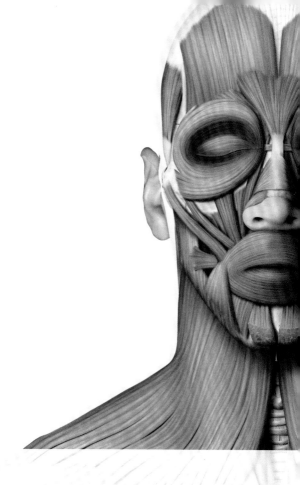

肌肉 Muscles

肌肉是主要由肌纤维组成的器官。在神经冲动的作用下，肌肉可以收缩。肌肉分布于人体全身，执行与运动相关的各种功能。人体最多的肌肉是骨骼肌，骨骼肌通过肌腱附着于骨骼。骨骼肌参与骨骼、舌头以及皮肤的复杂运动，并能产生肌张力。平滑肌负责血管以及很多空腔器官的运动活动。平滑肌的运动特征具有非特异性、节律性和渐进性。最后一种肌肉是心肌，心肌负责心脏的收缩。

Muscles are organs formed mainly of muscle fibres, which contract in reaction to nerve impulses. They are present throughout the body and perform various functions related to body movements. The most numerous are the skeletal muscles, attached to the skeleton by tendons. They generate the complex movements of bones, the tongue, and the skin, and are responsible for muscle tone. Smooth muscles are responsible for motor activity of the blood vessels and many hollow organs; their movements are nonspecific, rhythmic, or graduated. Finally, cardiac muscle is responsible for the heart's contractions.

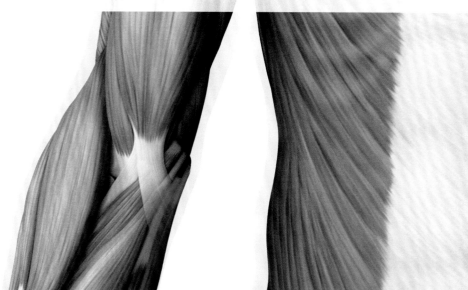

肌肉
主要由肌纤维组成的器官，可以在神经冲动的作用下产生收缩反应，可使人体运动和保持姿态。

muscle
Organ made up essentially of muscle fibers and having the ability to contract under the action of a nervous influx; muscles allow the body to move and maintain posture.

肌肉类型
肌肉分三种类型。每种都有各自的特性。

types of muscles
There are three types of muscles, each with specific characteristics.

平滑肌
能使特定器官产生非自主运动的肌肉。主要分布于空腔器官（如肠道和食管）的管壁和血管壁。

smooth muscle
Muscle allowing involuntary movements of certain organs; they are found mostly in the walls of hollow organs (such as the intestines and the esophagus) and blood vessels.

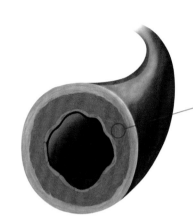

平滑肌纤维
只有单个细胞核的小型梭状肌细胞。

smooth muscle fiber
Small fusiform muscle cell having a single nucleus.

条纹状肌肉纤维
具有多个细胞核和特征性横纹的肌肉细胞。

striated muscle fiber
Muscle cell having numerous nuclei and characteristic transversal striation.

骨骼肌
通过肌腱附着于骨骼，在收缩时能使骨骼产生自主运动的肌肉。

skeletal muscle
Muscle that, when contracting, allows voluntary movements of the skeleton to which it is attached by tendons.

起点
骨骼上的骨骼肌附着点。骨骼肌收缩时，起点不会发生移动。

origin
Anchor point of the skeletal muscle on the bone that remains stable during muscle contraction.

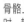

肌腹
骨骼肌的中间部分，位于起点和止点之间。

belly
Central part of a skeletal muscle, between the origin and the insertion

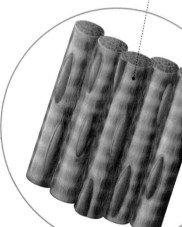

止点
骨骼上的骨骼肌附着点。骨骼肌收缩时，止点会发生移动。

insertion
Anchor point of the skeletal muscle on the bone that moves during muscle contraction.

肌腱
无弹性的纤维结缔组织束。位于骨骼肌末端，止于骨骼。

tendon
Band of inelastic fibrous connective tissue at the extreme end of a skeletal muscle, anchoring it on the bone.

心肌
构成心脏大部分的肌肉。由肌纤维支链组成，能使心脏收缩。

cardiac muscle
Muscle making up the largest part of the heart, formed of branching chains of muscle fibers; it allows the heart to contract.

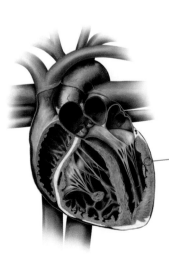

心肌纤维
有单个中央细胞核和横纹的肌肉细胞。

cardiac muscle fiber
Muscle cell with a single central nucleus and transversal striation.

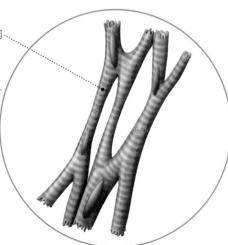

肌腱
无弹性的纤维结缔组织束。位于骨骼肌末端，止于骨骼。
tendon
Band of inelastic fibrous connective tissue at the extreme end of a skeletal muscle, anchoring it on the bone.

筋膜
疏松结缔组织膜。可在骨骼肌周围形成包膜，隔离周边其他组织。
fascia
Membrane of loose connective tissue forming an envelope around a skeletal muscle and isolating it from surrounding tissues.

肌肉组织
由细长可收缩细胞（称为肌纤维）构成的组织。
muscle tissue
Tissue made up of elongated contractile cells, the muscle fibers.

骨骼肌结构
structure of a skeletal muscle

肌肉
主要由肌纤维组成的器官。可在神经冲动的作用下收缩。
muscle
Organ made up mainly of muscle fiber, able to contract under the action of a nerve impulse.

肌纤维束
肌纤维群。
bundle of muscle fibers
Group of muscle fibers.

肌束膜
结缔组织。包裹肌纤维束。
perimysium
Layer of connective tissue surrounding a bundle of muscle fibers.

肌纤维
可收缩的细胞。组成肌肉。
muscle fiber
Contractile cell, constituent element of muscles.

运动神经元
能将中枢神经系统发出的神经冲动传导到肌肉的神经元。
motor neuron
Neuron transmitting nerve impulses from the central nervous system to the muscles.

肌膜
肌纤维的细胞膜。
sarcolemma
Cell membrane of a muscle fiber.

肌原纤维
长且具有收缩功能的肌丝。组成骨骼肌的肌纤维。肌丝主要由两种蛋白质（肌动蛋白和肌球蛋白）组成。
myofibril
Long contractile filament making up the muscle fibers of the skeletal muscles, consisting of two main proteins (actin and myosin).

重量可观 | Heavy Weight

人体的600多块骨骼肌约占人体总质量的一半。
Together, the some 600 skeletal muscles in the human body account for almost half of the body's total mass.

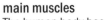

主要肌肉
人体全身分布着600多块肌肉。

main muscles
The human body has more than 600_muscles distributed throughout the body.

主要肌肉前面观
main muscles: anterior view

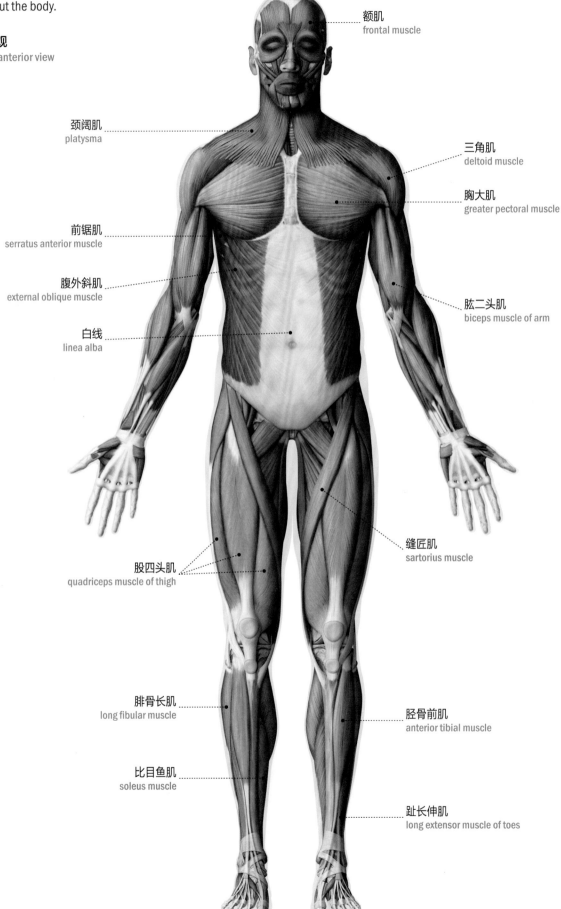

额肌
frontal muscle

颈阔肌
platysma

三角肌
deltoid muscle

胸大肌
greater pectoral muscle

前锯肌
serratus anterior muscle

腹外斜肌
external oblique muscle

肱二头肌
biceps muscle of arm

白线
linea alba

缝匠肌
sartorius muscle

股四头肌
quadriceps muscle of thigh

腓骨长肌
long fibular muscle

胫骨前肌
anterior tibial muscle

比目鱼肌
soleus muscle

趾长伸肌
long extensor muscle of toes

颈阔肌

成对肌肉。在下颌和锁骨之间，覆盖颈部前部，可使所有颈前皮肤向下颌牵拉。

platysma
Paired muscle covering the anterior face of the neck, between the chin and clavicle; it all of the chin to be drawn.

前锯肌

成对肌肉。将第1到第9肋骨连接至肩胛骨，尤可使肩胛骨外旋。

serratus anterior muscle
Paired muscle connecting the first nine ribs to the shoulder blade; it allows especially lateral rotation of the shoulder blade.

腹外斜肌

成对肌肉。将下位的8条肋骨连接到髂骨，可使躯干屈曲和旋转。包紧内脏器官。

external oblique muscle
Paired muscle connecting the last eight ribs to the iliac bone; it allows flexion and rotation of the trunk and compression of the internal organs.

白线

纤维性膜。沿着腹壁中线向下走行，作为某些腹部肌肉的止点。

linea alba
Fibrous membrane running down the midline of the abdominal wall, serving as an insertion point for some abdominal muscles.

股四头肌

成对肌肉。由四个头覆盖大腿前部，可使小腿伸展和大腿屈曲。

quadriceps muscle of thigh
Paired muscle with four heads forming the anterior part of the thigh; it allows extension of the leg and flexion of the thigh.

腓骨长肌

成对肌肉。将胫骨和腓骨连接到内侧楔骨和第一跖骨，辅助足部的多个动作，如外展、屈曲、外旋。

long fibular muscle
Paired muscle connecting the tibia and fibula with the medial cuneiform and first metatarsal bones; it assists in several movements of the foot (abduction, flexion, outward rotation).

比目鱼肌

成对肌肉。将胫骨和腓骨连接到跟骨，可使足部伸展，是行走和跑步的重要肌肉。

soleus muscle
Paired muscle connecting the tibia and fibula to the calcaneus; it allows extension of the foot, making it an important muscle for walking and running.

额肌

不成对的大块肌肉。连接眼眶上部和颅顶腱膜，可使前额皮肤皱起，上提眉毛。

frontal muscle
Large unpaired muscle connecting the upper part of the orbit and the epicranial aponeurosis; it allows the skin of the forehead to crease and the eyebrows to lift.

三角肌

成对肌肉。覆盖锁骨，肩胛骨和肱骨之间的肩部，能辅助手臂的多个动作，如外展，屈曲，伸展。

deltoid muscle
Paired muscle covering the shoulder between the clavicle, shoulder blade and humerus; it assists in several movements of the arm (abduction, flexion, extension).

胸大肌

成对肌肉。将胸骨和锁骨连接到肱骨，尤其可使手臂外旋以及向身体的轴线方向移动，即内收。

greater pectoral muscle
Paired muscle connecting the sternum and clavicle to the humerus; it allows especially the arm to rotate outward and to move toward the axis of the body (adduction).

肱二头肌

成对肌肉。由两个头组成，连接肩胛骨与桡骨，可使前臂屈曲和外旋。

biceps muscle of arm
Paired muscle formed of two heads, connecting the shoulder blade to the radius; it allows flexion and outward rotation of the forearm

缝匠肌

成对肌肉。连接髂骨与胫骨，可使大腿屈曲和旋转，小腿屈曲。

sartorius muscle
Paired muscle connecting the iliac bone to the tibia; it allows flexion and rotation of the thigh, as well as flexion of the leg.

胫骨前肌

成对肌肉。将胫骨连接到内侧楔骨和第一跖骨，可使足部屈曲并向身体的轴线方向移动。

anterior tibial muscle
Paired muscle connecting the tibia to the medial cuneiform and first metatarsal bones; it allows the foot to flex and move toward the axis of the body.

趾长伸肌

成对肌肉。将腓骨和胫骨外侧髁连接到四个外侧足趾，可使足趾伸展。

long extensor muscle of toes
Pired muscle connecting the fibula and lateral condyle of the tibia to the last four toes, allowing them to extend.

肌肉 | MUSCLES

主要肌肉后面观
main muscles: posterior view

枕肌
occipital muscle

胸锁乳突肌
sternocleidomastoid muscle

斜方肌
trapezius muscle

三角肌
deltoid muscle

冈下肌
infraspinatus muscle

大圆肌
teres major muscle

肱三头肌
triceps muscle of arm

背阔肌
latissimus dorsi muscle

臀大肌
gluteus maximus muscle

大收肌
great adductor muscle

半腱肌
semitendinous muscle

股二头肌
biceps muscle of thigh

半膜肌
semimembranous muscle

腓肠肌
gastrocnemius muscle

跟腱
calcaneal tendon

多种多样的肌肉 | A Wide Diversity

人体肌肉形态各异，大小不一。最长的肌肉是大腿部的缝匠肌，最宽的是腹外斜肌。

The body's muscles have a wide variety of shapes and sizes. The longest muscle is the sartorius, in the thigh, while the widest is the external oblique muscle of abdomen.

枕肌

不成对肌肉。连接枕骨和帽状腱膜，可使头皮后拉。

occipital muscle
Unpaired muscle connecting the occipital bone to the epicranial aponeurosis; it allows the scalp to pull back.

斜方肌

成对三角形肌肉。连接枕骨、相应椎骨到锁骨、肩峰和肩胛骨，可使肩关节活动及协助头部后仰。

trapezius muscle
Triangular paired muscle connecting the occipital bone and certain vertebrae to the clavicle, acromion and shoulder blade; it allows numerous movements of the shoulder and assists in the extension of the head

冈下肌

成对肌肉。连接肩胛骨和肱骨，主要使手臂外旋。

infraspinatus muscle
Paired muscle connecting the shoulder blade to the humerus; it allows mainly outward rotation of the arm.

大圆肌

成对肌肉。连接肩胛骨和肱骨，可使手臂内旋，并向身体的轴线移动（内收）。

teres major muscle
Paired muscle connecting the shoulder blade to the humerus; it allows the arm to rotate inward and to move toward the axis of the body (adduction).

背阔肌

大块扁平成对肌肉。连接脊柱与肱骨，可使手臂内旋并向身体轴线方向移动（内收）。

latissimus dorsi muscle
Large, flat paired muscle connecting the vertebral column to the humerus; it allows the arm to rotate inward and to move toward the axis of the body (adduction).

大收肌

成对肌肉。连接耻骨与股骨，可使大腿向身体的轴线方向移动（内收）、外旋、屈曲和伸展。

great adductor muscle
Paired muscle connecting the pubis to the femur; it allows the thigh to move toward the axis of the body (adduction), rotate outward, flex and extend.

半膜肌

成对肌肉。连接坐骨到胫骨和股骨，可使小腿屈曲和内旋，大腿伸展。

semimembranous muscle
Paired muscle connecting the ischium to the tibia and femur; it allows flexion and inward rotation of the leg, and extension of the thigh.

腓肠肌

成对肌肉。连接股骨和跟骨，由两个头组成。可使足部和小腿屈曲。

gastrocnemius muscle
Paired muscle formed of two heads connecting the femur to the calcaneus; it allows flexion of the foot and leg.

胸锁乳突肌

成对肌肉。由两个头组成，连接颞骨至胸骨和锁骨，可使头部屈曲、侧倾和旋转。

sternocleidomastoid muscle
Paired muscle formed of two heads, connecting the temporal bone to the manubrium and clavicle; it allows flexion, lateral inclination and rotation of the head.

三角肌

成对肌肉。覆盖在锁骨，肩胛骨和肱骨之间的肩部。其可使手臂外展，屈曲，伸展。

deltoid muscle
Paired muscle covering the shoulder between the clavicle, shoulder blade and humerus; it assists in several movements of the arm (abduction, flexion, extension).

肱三头肌

成对肌肉。由三个头组成，连接肩胛骨、肱骨和尺骨鹰嘴。构成手臂的后表面，可使前臂伸展。

triceps muscle of arm
Paired muscle formed of three heads connecting the shoulder blade and humerus to the olecranon, forming the posterior face of the arm; it allows extension of the forearm.

臀大肌

成对肌肉。构成臀部，保持躯干直立，可使髋关节伸展和外旋。

gluteus maximus muscle
Paired muscle forming the buttock, maintaining the trunk in an upright position and allowing extension and outward rotation of the hip.

半腱肌

成对肌肉。连接坐骨和胫骨，可使小腿屈曲和内旋，大腿伸展。

semitendinous muscle
Paired muscle connecting the ischium to the tibia; it allows flexion and inward rotation of the leg, as well as extension of the thigh.

股二头肌

成对肌肉。由两个头组成，连接股骨和坐骨至腓骨，可协助小腿屈曲。

biceps muscle of thigh
Paired muscle formed of two heads, connecting the femur and ischium to the fibula; it assists in bending the leg.

跟腱

踝关节后方的大型肌腱，连接小腿三头肌与跟骨。

calcaneal tendon
Large tendon of the posterior face of the ankle, connecting the triceps surae to the calcaneus.

头和颈 | head and neck

头和颈

头颈部包含面部肌肉（负责面部表情）和咀嚼肌。

head and neck

The head and neck contain especially the facial muscles (responsible for facial expressions) and the masticating muscles.

头颈部前面观
head and neck: anterior view

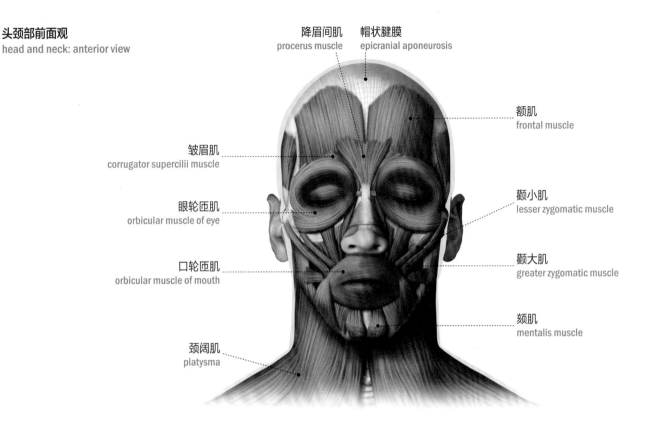

降眉间肌
procerus muscle

帽状腱膜
epicranial aponeurosis

额肌
frontal muscle

皱眉肌
corrugator supercilii muscle

颧小肌
lesser zygomatic muscle

眼轮匝肌
orbicular muscle of eye

颧大肌
greater zygomatic muscle

口轮匝肌
orbicular muscle of mouth

颏肌
mentalis muscle

颈阔肌
platysma

丰富的情感 | A Range of Emotions

面部表情由头部的70多块肌肉完成。全球统计的人类表情可细分为7 000种，其中有六种基本表情：喜悦、愤怒、恐惧、惊讶、厌恶和悲伤。

Facial expressions are formed by some 70 muscles in the head. There are six basic expressions-joy, anger, fear, surprise, disgust, and sadness-among the 7,000 physiognomies classified worldwide.

头颈部侧面观
head and neck: lateral view

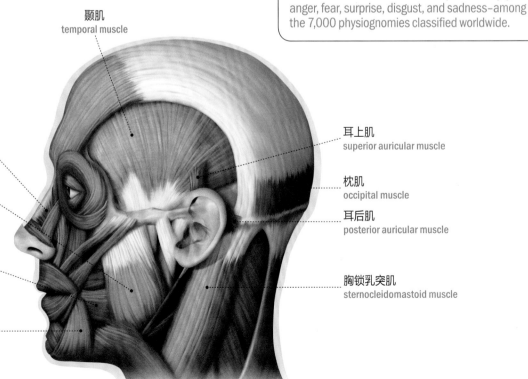

颞肌
temporal muscle

鼻肌
nasal muscle

咀嚼肌
masseter muscle

笑肌
risorius muscle

降口角肌
depressor muscle of angle of mouth

耳上肌
superior auricular muscle

枕肌
occipital muscle

耳后肌
posterior auricular muscle

胸锁乳突肌
sternocleidomastoid muscle

降眉间肌

不成对肌肉。连接鼻骨与前额皮肤，可下拉眉间的皮肤。

procerus muscle
Unpaired muscle connecting the nasal bone to the skin of the forehead; it allows the skin between the eyebrows to be pulled downward.

皱眉肌

小块成对肌肉。位于眼眶上方，可使眉毛抬起，额头皮肤皱起。

corrugator supercilii muscle
Small, paired muscle above the orbit, allowing the eyebrows to raise and the skin of the forehead to crease.

眼轮匝肌

环状成对肌肉。围绕眼眶并延伸到眼睑中，可控制眼睑和眼部周围的运动。

orbicular muscle of eye
Paired, ring-shaped muscle surrounding the orbit and extending into the eyelids; it controls the movements of the eyelids and periphery of the eye.

口轮匝肌

不成对肌肉。由两束组成，连接嘴角，可使嘴巴张开与闭合。

orbicular muscle of mouth
Unpaired muscle having two bundles connecting the corners of the lips, allowing the mouth to open and close especially.

颈阔肌

成对肌肉。分布于颈前部表面，位于下颚和锁骨之间。可提拉下颌皮肤。

platysma
Paired muscle covering the anterior face of the neck, between the chin and clavicle; it allows the skin of the chin to be drawn.

颞肌

成对肌肉。连接颞窝和下颌骨，可通过抬起下颌骨来关闭下颚。

temporal muscle
Paired muscle connecting the temporal fossa to the mandible; it allows the jaws to be closed by lifting the mandible.

鼻肌

成对肌肉。连接上颌骨和鼻梁骨，可使鼻孔扩张，鼻软骨降低。

nasal muscle
Paired muscle connecting the maxilla to the bridge of the nose; it allows the nostrils to be dilated and the cartilage of the nose to be lowered.

咀嚼肌

强力的成对肌肉。连接颧骨到下颌骨，可提拉颌骨的上部，实现咀嚼。

masseter muscle
Powerful paired muscle connecting the zygomatic bone to the mandible; it allows the upper jaw to be raised, contributing to chewing.

笑肌

成对肌肉。从咬肌延伸到嘴角，尤可产生微笑。

risorius muscle
Paired muscle extending from the masseter muscle to the angle of the mouth; it especially allows smiling.

降口角肌

成对肌肉。连接下颌骨和嘴角，可使嘴角下拉。

depressor muscle of angle of mouth
Paired muscle connecting the mandible to the angle of the mouth, allowing it to be lowered.

帽状腱膜

纤维层。覆盖颅骨，位于额肌和枕肌之间。

epicranial aponeurosis
Fibrous layer covering the skull, between the frontal and occipital muscles.

额肌

大块的不成对肌肉。连接眼眶上部和帽状腱膜，可皱起前额的皮肤，上提眉毛。

frontal muscle
Large, unpaired muscle connecting the upper part of the orbit and the epicranial aponeurosis; it allows the skin of the forehead to crease and the eyebrows to lift.

颧小肌

连接颧骨与嘴角的成对肌肉，可协助微笑。

lesser zygomatic muscle
Paired muscle connecting the zygomatic bone to the upper lip; it assists in smiling.

颧大肌

连接颧骨和上唇的成对肌肉，可协助微笑。

greater zygomatic muscle
Paired muscle connecting the zygomatic bone to the angle of the mouth; it assists in smiling.

颏肌

小块成对肌肉。连接下颏的骨和皮肤，收缩可抬起下颏。

mentalis muscle
Small, paired muscle connecting the bone and skin of the chin; its contraction allows the chin to be raised.

耳上肌

成对肌肉。连接帽状腱膜至耳部软骨，可稍微上提耳部。

superior auricular muscle
Paired muscle connecting the epicranial aponeurosis to the cartilage of the ear; it pulls the ear slightly upward.

枕肌

成对肌肉。连接枕骨和帽状腱膜，可后拉头皮。

occipital muscle
Paired muscle connecting the occipital bone to the epicranial aponeurosis; it allows the scalp to be pulled back.

耳后肌

成对肌肉。连接乳突至耳部软骨，可把耳朵向上和向后稍微拉动。

posterior auricular muscle
Paired muscle connecting the mastoid apophysis to the cartilage of the ear; it pulls the ear slightly up and back.

胸锁乳突肌

成对肌肉。由两个头组成，连接颞骨到胸骨和锁骨，可使头部屈曲、侧倾和旋转。

sternocleidomastoid muscle
Paired muscle formed of two heads, connecting the temporal bone to the manubrium and clavicle; it allows flexion, lateral inclination and rotation of the head.

胸腹部 | thorax and abdomen

胸腹部

胸廓和腹壁包含具有支撑功能的腹部浅层和深层肌肉，可使躯干和四肢能够完成多种运动。

thorax and abdomen

The thoracic cage and abdominal wall contain superficial and deep muscles that support the abdomen and enable the trunk and limbs to perform numerous movements.

胸腹部前面观
thorax and abdomen: anterior view

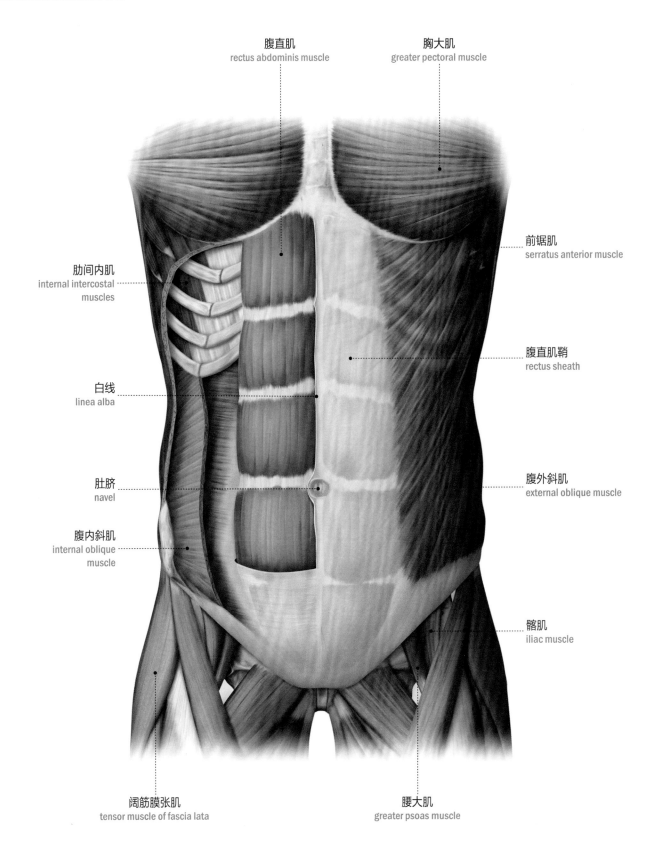

腹直肌
rectus abdominis muscle

胸大肌
greater pectoral muscle

前锯肌
serratus anterior muscle

肋间内肌
internal intercostal muscles

腹直肌鞘
rectus sheath

白线
linea alba

肚脐
navel

腹外斜肌
external oblique muscle

腹内斜肌
internal oblique muscle

髂肌
iliac muscle

阔筋膜张肌
tensor muscle of fascia lata

腰大肌
greater psoas muscle

腹直肌

不成对的腹部浅表肌肉。连接耻骨至胸骨和某些肋软骨。主要能使躯干前屈。

rectus abdominis muscle
Unpaired, superficial muscle of the abdomen connecting the pubis to the sternum and certain costal cartilages; it allows especially forward flexion of the trunk.

胸大肌

成对的双头肌肉。连接胸骨、锁骨至肱骨。可使手臂拉近身体（内收），更主要的是能使手臂外旋。

greater pectoral muscle
Paired muscle formed of two heads, connecting the sternum and clavicle to the humerus; it allows especially the arm to rotate outward, as well as to draw close to the body (adduction).

肋间内肌

成对肌肉。连接肋骨下缘和下位肋骨上缘。呼气时肌肉活动，可下拉肋骨。

internal intercostal muscles
Paired muscles connecting the lower border of one rib to the upper border of the underlying rib; active during exhalation, it allows especially the ribs to be lowered.

前锯肌

成对肌肉。连接上位九根肋骨和肩胛骨，尤可使肩胛骨外旋，从而协助手臂外展。

serratus anterior muscle
Paired muscle connecting the first nine ribs to the shoulder blade; it allows especially lateral rotation of the shoulder blade, thus assisting in the abduction of the arm.

白线

纤维膜。沿腹壁中线向下延伸走行。可作为某些腹部肌肉的止点。

linea alba
Fibrous membrane running down the midline of the abdominal wall, serving as an insertion point for some abdominal muscles.

腹直肌鞘

覆盖腹直肌的膜。其内侧缘参与形成白线。

rectus sheath
Membrane covering the rectus muscle of the abdomen; its inner border assists the formation of the linea alba.

肚脐

圆形凹陷疤痕。由脐带切断后形成。

navel
Scar in the form of a rounded depression resulting from the cutting of the umbilical cord.

腹外斜肌

大而薄的成对肌肉。连接下位八根肋骨和髂骨，可使躯干屈曲和旋转，包紧支撑内脏并有助于呼气。

external oblique muscle
Large, thin paired muscle connecting the last eight ribs to the iliac bone; it allows flexion and rotation of the trunk and compression of the internal organs and contributes to exhalation.

腹内斜肌

成对肌肉。连接髂骨至最后三或四根肋骨，除了能包紧支撑内脏，还可使躯干屈曲和旋转。

internal oblique muscle
Paired muscle connecting the iliac bone to the last three or four ribs; it allows flexion and rotation of the trunk, as well as compression of the internal organs.

髂肌

成对肌肉。位于下腹部，主要可使大腿屈曲。

iliac muscle
Paired muscle of the lower region of the abdomen that allows mainly flexion of the thigh.

阔筋膜张肌

成对肌肉。连接髂骨和大腿周围膜（阔筋膜）的边缘，有助于髋关节的屈曲和内旋。

tensor muscle of fascia lata
Paired muscle connecting the iliac bone to the edge of the membrane surrounding the thigh (fascia lata); it contributes to flexion and inward rotation of the hip.

腰大肌

成对肌肉。可使大腿屈曲或躯干向前弯曲。

greater psoas muscle
Paired muscle that allows flexion of the thigh or forward bending of the trunk.

上肢

肩、上臂、前臂和手包含许多块肌肉，可做出十分精细的动作。

upper limb

The shoulder, arm, forearm and hand contain numerous muscles that allow movements of great precision.

上肢前面观
upper limb: anterior view

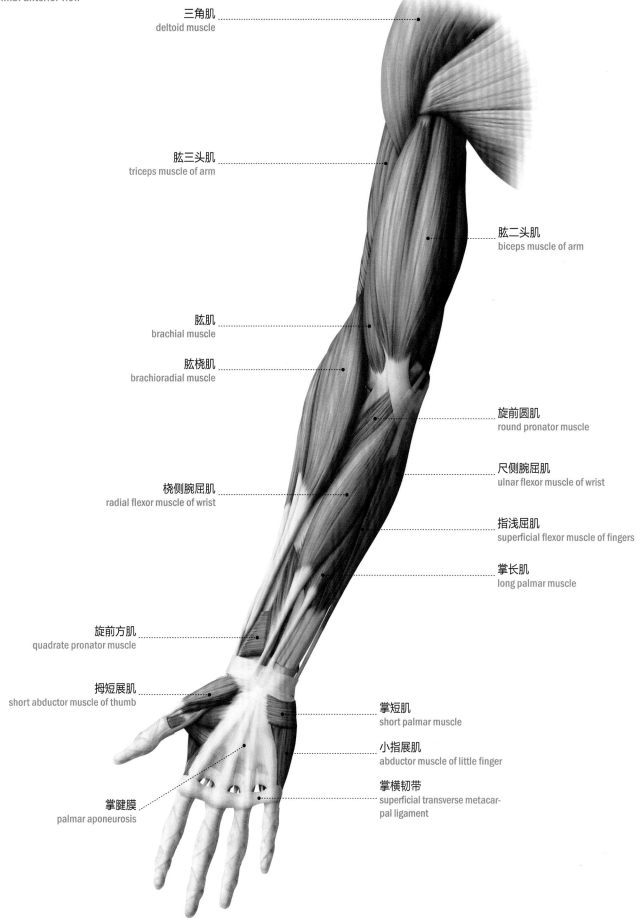

三角肌
deltoid muscle

肱三头肌
triceps muscle of arm

肱二头肌
biceps muscle of arm

肱肌
brachial muscle

肱桡肌
brachioradial muscle

旋前圆肌
round pronator muscle

尺侧腕屈肌
ulnar flexor muscle of wrist

桡侧腕屈肌
radial flexor muscle of wrist

指浅屈肌
superficial flexor muscle of fingers

掌长肌
long palmar muscle

旋前方肌
quadrate pronator muscle

拇短展肌
short abductor muscle of thumb

掌短肌
short palmar muscle

小指展肌
abductor muscle of little finger

掌横韧带
superficial transverse metacarpal ligament

掌腱膜
palmar aponeurosis

三角肌

覆盖锁骨、肩胛骨和肱骨的肩部肌肉。协助上臂外展，屈曲，伸展。

deltoid muscle
Muscle covering the shoulder between the clavicle, shoulder blade and humerus; it assists in several movements of the arm (abduction, flexion, extension).

肱三头肌

连接肩胛骨、肱骨至尺骨鹰嘴的肌肉。覆盖上臂的后面，可使前臂伸展。

triceps muscle of arm
Muscle connecting the shoulder blade and humerus to the olecranon, forming the posterior face of the arm; it allows extension of the forearm.

肱肌

连接肱骨和尺骨的肌肉。可使前臂屈曲。

brachial muscle
Muscle connecting the humerus to the ulna; it allows flexion of the forearm.

肱桡肌

连接肱骨至桡骨外侧面的肌肉。可使前臂屈曲，协助其外旋。

brachioradial muscle
Muscle connecting the humerus to the lateral face of the radius; it allows flexion of the forearm and assists in its outward rotation.

桡侧腕屈肌

连接肱骨和第二掌骨的肌肉。可使手部弯曲和移开身体轴线（外展）。

radial flexor muscle of wrist
Muscle connecting the humerus to the second metacarpal; it allows the hand to flex and move away from the axis of the body (abduction).

旋前方肌

连接尺骨和桡骨的肌肉。可使前臂内旋（旋前）。

quadrate pronator muscle
Muscle connecting the ulna to the radius, allowing inward rotation of the forearm (pronation).

拇短展肌

连接大多角骨和拇指近节指骨的浅部肌肉。可使拇指移开手部轴线方向（外展）。

short abductor muscle of thumb
Superficial muscle connecting the trapezium bone to the proximal phalanx of the thumb; it mainly allows the thumb to move away from the axis of the hand (abduction).

掌腱膜

连接手指屈肌肌腱的三角形筋膜。

palmar aponeurosis
Triangular-shaped membrane connecting the tendons of the flexor muscles of the fingers.

肱二头肌

双头肌肉。连接肩胛骨和桡骨，可使前臂屈曲和外旋。

biceps muscle of arm
Muscle formed of two heads, connecting the shoulder blade to the radius; it allows flexion and outward rotation of the forearm.

旋前圆肌

双头肌肉。连接肱骨、尺骨至桡骨，可使前臂屈曲和内旋（旋前）。

round pronator muscle
Muscle formed of two heads, connecting the humerus and ulna to the radius; it allows flexion and inward rotation (pronation) of the forearm.

尺侧腕屈肌

双头肌肉。连接肱骨、尺骨到豌豆骨，可使手部屈曲并向身体轴线方向移动（内收）。

ulnar flexor muscle of wrist
Muscle having two heads, connecting the humerus and ulna to the pisiform bone; it allows the hand to flex and move toward the axis of the body (adduction).

指浅屈肌

双头肌肉。连接肱骨、尺骨和桡骨至手指的中节指骨，可使后四根手指屈曲。

superficial flexor muscle of fingers
Muscle having two heads, connecting the humerus, ulna and radius to the middle phalanges of the fingers; it allows mainly flexion of the last four fingers.

掌长肌

连接肱骨到掌腱膜的肌肉。可使腕关节屈曲。

long palmar muscle
Muscle connecting the humerus to the palmar aponeurosis; it allows flexion of the wrist.

掌短肌

连接掌腱膜和手内侧缘皮肤的肌肉。可牵拉手掌的部分皮肤折起出现褶皱。

short palmar muscle
Muscle connecting the palmar aponeurosis to the skin of the inside edge of the hand; it allows the skin of part of the palm to be folded.

小指展肌

连接大多角骨和小指近节指骨的肌肉。可使小指从手部轴线方向外移（外展）。

abductor muscle of little finger
Muscle connecting the pisiform bone to the proximal phalanx of the little finger, allowing it to move away from the axis of the hand (abduction).

掌横韧带

位于掌腱膜底层的韧带。

superficial transverse metacarpal ligament
Ligament at the base of the palmar aponeurosis.

手后面观
hand: posterior view

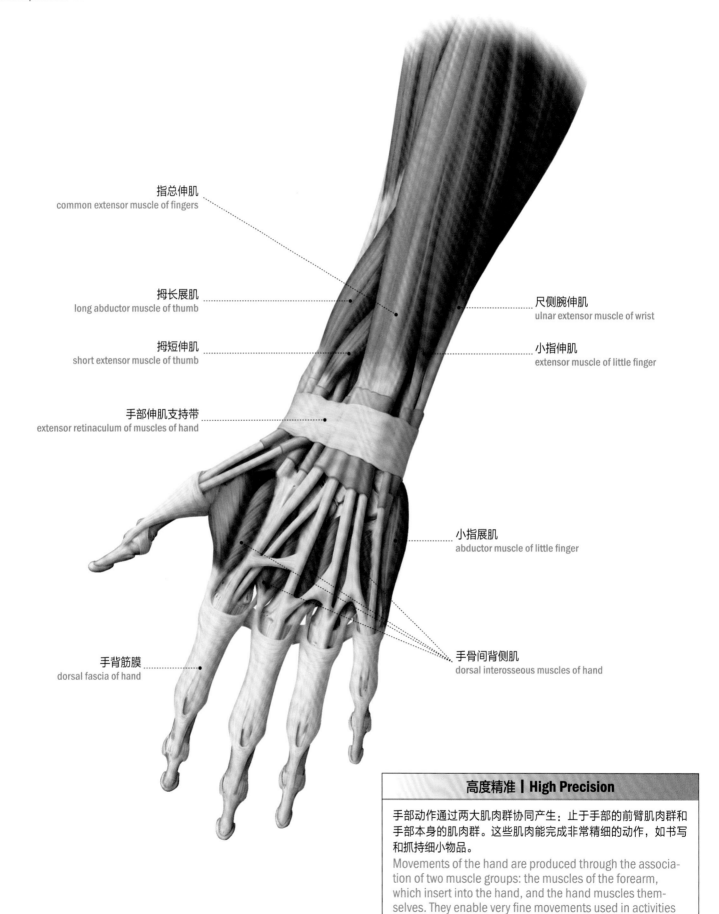

指总伸肌
common extensor muscle of fingers

拇长展肌
long abductor muscle of thumb

拇短伸肌
short extensor muscle of thumb

手部伸肌支持带
extensor retinaculum of muscles of hand

尺侧腕伸肌
ulnar extensor muscle of wrist

小指伸肌
extensor muscle of little finger

小指展肌
abductor muscle of little finger

手骨间背侧肌
dorsal interosseous muscles of hand

手背筋膜
dorsal fascia of hand

高度精准 | High Precision

手部动作通过两大肌肉群协同产生：止于手部的前臂肌肉群和手部本身的肌肉群。这些肌肉能完成非常精细的动作，如书写和抓持细小物品。

Movements of the hand are produced through the association of two muscle groups: the muscles of the forearm, which insert into the hand, and the hand muscles themselves. They enable very fine movements used in activities such as writing and gripping delicate objects.

指总伸肌
连接肱骨至后四指的中节和远节指骨的肌肉。可使手指伸展（除外拇指），并辅助手部伸展。

common extensor muscle of fingers
Muscle connecting the humerus to the middle and distal phalanges of the last four fingers; it allows extension of the fingers (except the thumb) and assists in extension of the hand.

拇长展肌
连接桡骨和尺骨至第一掌骨的肌肉。可使拇指伸展并移开手部轴线方向（外展）。

long abductor muscle of thumb
Muscle connecting the radius and the ulna to the first metacarpal; it allows the thumb to extend and to move away from the axis of the hand (abduction).

拇短伸肌
连接桡骨至拇指近节指骨的肌肉。可使拇指伸展并远离手部轴线方向（外展）。

short extensor muscle of thumb
Muscle connecting the radius to the proximal phalanx of the thumb; it allows the thumb to extend and to move away from the axis of the hand (abduction).

手部伸肌支持带
覆盖手部伸肌肌腱的纤维层。

extensor retinaculum of muscles of hand
Fibrous layer covering the tendons of the extensor muscles of the hand.

手背筋膜
由伸肌的支持带延长而来的手背纤维膜。

dorsal fascia of hand
Fibrous membrane of the back of the hand, prolonged by the retinaculum of the extensor muscles.

尺侧腕伸肌
连接肱骨、尺骨至第五掌骨的肌肉。可使手部向后弯曲（伸展）并向身体的轴线移动（内收）。

ulnar extensor muscle of wrist
Muscle connecting the humerus and ulna to the fifth metacarpal; it allows the hand to fold backward (extension) and to move toward the axis of the body (adduction).

小指伸肌
连接肱骨和小指的肌肉。可使小指伸展。

extensor muscle of little finger
Muscle connecting the humerus to the little finger, allowing it to extend.

小指展肌
连接豌豆骨和小指近节指骨的肌肉。可使小指移开手部轴线（外展）。

abductor muscle of little finger
Muscle connecting the pisiform bone to the proximal phalanx of the little finger, allowing it to move away from the axis of the hand (abduction).

手骨间背侧肌
连接掌骨至后四指的近节指骨的肌肉。可使后四指弯曲和分开。

dorsal interosseous muscles of hand
Muscles connecting the metacarpals to the proximal phalanges of the last four fingers; it allows the fingers to bend and to spread apart.

下肢

大腿、小腿和足包含很多肌肉，可使人体保持站立和移动。

lower limb

The thigh, leg and foot contain numerous muscles that allow upright stance and locomotion.

下肢前面观
lower limb: anterior view

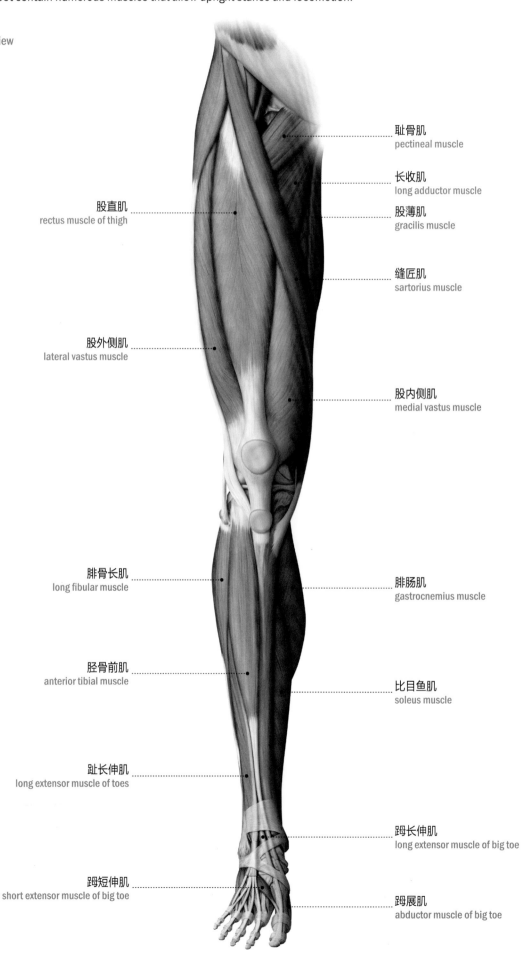

耻骨肌
pectineal muscle

长收肌
long adductor muscle

股直肌
rectus muscle of thigh

股薄肌
gracilis muscle

缝匠肌
sartorius muscle

股外侧肌
lateral vastus muscle

股内侧肌
medial vastus muscle

腓骨长肌
long fibular muscle

腓肠肌
gastrocnemius muscle

胫骨前肌
anterior tibial muscle

比目鱼肌
soleus muscle

趾长伸肌
long extensor muscle of toes

蹞长伸肌
long extensor muscle of big toe

蹞短伸肌
short extensor muscle of big toe

蹞展肌
abductor muscle of big toe

股直肌

股四头肌的中央部分。将髂骨和髋臼连接到髌骨和胫骨，可使小腿伸展和大腿屈曲。

rectus muscle of thigh
Central part of the quadriceps, connecting the iliac bone and acetabulum to the patella and tibia; it allows extension of the leg and flexion of the thigh.

股外侧肌

股四头肌的一部分。与股骨外侧相连，可辅助小腿伸展和稳定膝关节。

lateral vastus muscle
Part of the quadriceps connected to the outer part of the femur; it assists the leg to extend and stabilizes the knee.

腓骨长肌

连接胫骨和腓骨至内侧楔骨及第一跖骨的肌肉。可使足部外展、屈曲和外旋。

long fibular muscle
Muscle connecting the tibia and fibula with the medial cuneiform and first metatarsal bones; it assists in several movements of the foot (abduction, flexion, outward rotation).

胫骨前肌

连接胫骨至内侧楔骨及第一跖骨的肌肉。可使足部弯曲并向身体轴线方向移动。

anterior tibial muscle
Muscle connecting the tibia to the medial cuneiform and first metatarsal bones; it allows the foot to flex and move toward the axis of the body.

趾长伸肌

连接胫骨和腓骨至后四足趾的肌肉。可使后四足趾伸展。

long extensor muscle of toes
Muscle connecting the fibula and tibia to the last four toes, allowing them to extend.

踇短伸肌

连接跟骨至踇趾近节指骨的肌肉。可使大脚趾伸展。

short extensor muscle of big toe
Muscle connecting the calcaneus to the proximal phalanx of the big toe, allowing it to extend.

耻骨肌

连接耻骨与股骨上部的肌肉。可辅助大腿屈曲并向身体轴线移动（内收）。

pectineal muscle
Muscle connecting the pubis to the upper part of the femur; it assists the thigh to flex and move toward the axis of the body (adduction).

长内收肌

连接耻骨与股骨的肌肉。可使大腿向身体的轴线移动（内收），外旋和屈曲。

long adductor muscle
Muscle connecting the pubis to the femur; it allows the thigh to move toward the axis of the body (adduction) and ensures its outward rotation and flexion.

股薄肌

连接耻骨与胫骨的肌肉。可使大腿向身体的轴线移动（内收），以及小腿屈曲和内旋。

gracilis muscle
Muscle connecting the pubis to the tibia; it allows the thigh to move toward the axis of the body (adduction), as well as flexion and inward rotation of the leg.

缝匠肌

连接髂骨和胫骨的肌肉。可使大腿屈曲和旋转，小腿屈曲。

sartorius muscle
Muscle connecting the iliac bone to the tibia; it allows flexion and rotation of the thigh, as well as flexion of the leg.

股内侧肌

股四头肌的一部分。与股骨内侧相连，可使小腿伸展和稳定膝关节。

medial vastus muscle
Part of the quadriceps connected to the inner part of the femur; it allows the leg to extend and stabilizes the knee.

腓肠肌

双头肌肉。连接股骨至跟骨，可使足部和小腿屈曲。

gastrocnemius muscle
Muscle formed of two heads connecting the femur to the calcaneus; it allows flexion of the foot and leg.

比目鱼肌

连接胫骨和腓骨至跟骨的肌肉。可使足部伸展，是行走和跑步的重要肌肉。

soleus muscle
Muscle connecting the tibia and fibula to the calcaneus; it allows extension of the foot, making it an important muscle for walking and running.

踇长伸肌

连接胫骨至踇趾远节趾骨的肌肉。可使大脚趾伸展和足部前曲。

long extensor muscle of big toe
Muscle connecting the tibia to the distal phalanx of the big toe; it allows extension of the big toe and forward flexion of the foot.

踇展肌

连接跟骨至踇趾近节指骨的肌肉。可使大脚趾屈曲并移开足部轴线方向（外展）。

abductor muscle of big toe
Muscle connecting the calcaneus to the proximal phalanx of the big toe; it allows the big toe to flex and move away from the axis of the foot (abduction).

足侧面观
foot: lateral view

平衡点 | Balance Point

每足共有33块肌肉，其中部分足肌上达于腿部骨骼之间。足肌有助于维持身体平衡，并对行走发挥关键作用。

Each foot contains 33 muscles, some of which are inserted into the leg bones. They contribute to maintenance of balance and play an essential role in walking.

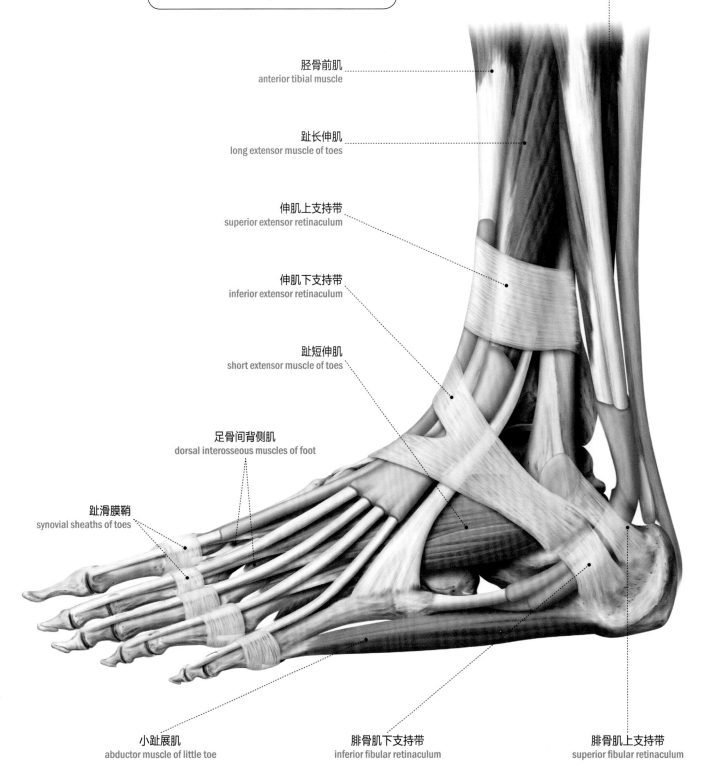

腓骨短肌
short fibular muscle

胫骨前肌
anterior tibial muscle

趾长伸肌
long extensor muscle of toes

伸肌上支持带
superior extensor retinaculum

伸肌下支持带
inferior extensor retinaculum

趾短伸肌
short extensor muscle of toes

足骨间背侧肌
dorsal interosseous muscles of foot

趾滑膜鞘
synovial sheaths of toes

小趾展肌
abductor muscle of little toe

腓骨肌下支持带
inferior fibular retinaculum

腓骨肌上支持带
superior fibular retinaculum

胫骨前肌

将胫骨连接至内侧楔骨和第一跖骨的肌肉。可使足部屈曲和移向身体轴线方向。

anterior tibial muscle
Muscle connecting the tibia to the medial cuneiform and first metatarsal bones; it allows the foot to flex and move toward the axis of the body.

趾长伸肌

连接胫腓骨和后四个足趾的肌肉。可使后四足趾伸展。

long extensor muscle of toes
Muscle connecting the fibula and tibia to the last four toes, allowing them to extend.

伸肌上支持带

位于踝关节上方的韧带。在足部活动过程中固定肌腱。

superior extensor retinaculum
Ligament above the ankle, anchoring the muscle tendons during movements of the foot.

伸肌下支持带

位于踝关节的前表面的韧带。两踝之间，在足部活动过程中固定肌腱。

inferior extensor retinaculum
Ligament of the anterior face of the ankle, between the two malleoli, anchoring the muscle tendons during movements of the foot.

趾短伸肌

连接跟骨与足趾的肌肉。可使足趾伸展。

short extensor muscle of toes
Muscle connecting the calcaneus to the toes, allowing them to extend.

足骨间背侧肌

连接跖骨和后四个足趾近节趾骨的肌肉。可使足趾屈曲以及彼此分开。

dorsal interosseous muscles of foot
Muscles connecting the metatarsals to the proximal phalanges of the last four toes; it allows the toes to flex and spread from each other.

趾滑膜鞘

覆盖趾伸肌腱的滑膜。

synovial sheaths of toes
Synovial membranes covering the flexor tendons of the toes.

腓骨短肌

连接腓骨和第五跖骨的肌肉。可使足部屈曲和旋转。

short fibular muscle
Muscle connecting the fibula to the fifth metatarsal; it allows flexion and rotation of the foot.

腓骨肌上支持带

从外踝延伸到跟骨的韧带。将腓骨长短肌固定在足的外侧。

superior fibular retinaculum
Ligament extending from the lateral malleolus to the calcaneus, anchoring the long and short fibular muscles to the outer face of the foot.

腓骨肌下支持带

从跟骨延伸到伸肌支持带的韧带。将腓骨长短肌固定到足的外侧。

inferior fibular retinaculum
Ligament extending from the calcaneus to the retinaculum of the extensor muscles, anchoring the long and short fibular muscles to the outer face of the foot.

小趾展肌

连接跟骨至小脚趾近节指骨的肌肉。可使小脚趾移开足部轴线方向（外展）。

abductor muscle of little toe
Muscle connecting the calcaneus to the proximal phalanx of the little toe; it allows the little toe to move away from the axis of the foot (abduction).

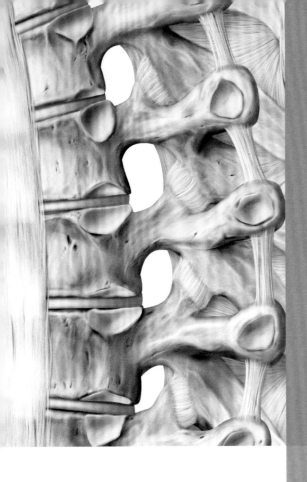

关节 Joints

关节是具有不同灵活程度的结构。关节把骨骼连在一起成为骨架，使其既稳固又灵活。骨骼的活动范围在很大程度上取决于其关节特性。纤维关节和软骨关节的活动范围很小，而滑膜关节的活动范围则很大。人体的滑膜关节有几百个，其中对身体活动最重要的关节分布在四肢和脊柱。

The joints are structures with varying degrees of mobility; they link bones together and provide the skeleton with solidity and mobility. A bone's range of motion depends in large part on the nature of its joints. Fibrous and cartilaginous joints have very little mobility, while synovial joints allow a wide variety of movements. Among the hundreds of synovial joints in the human body, the most important for mobility are those in the limbs and the spine.

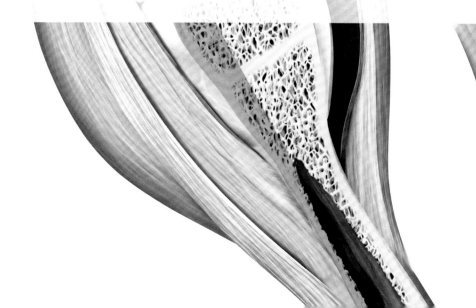

主要关节
关节主要分为三种类型：滑膜关节、软骨关节和纤维关节。

main joints
Joints are classified into three main types: synovial, cartilaginous and fibrous.

滑膜关节
此类关节的特征是具有关节囊，囊内充满黏性液体（滑液）。滑膜关节是最常见的一种关节。

synovial joints
Joints characterized by the presence of an articular capsule filled with viscous fluid (synovia); these are the most common joints.

软骨关节
其软骨板与关节表面融合在一起，灵活度有限。

cartilaginous joints
Joints having a cartilage plate fused with the articular surfaces; they allow only limited movement.

纤维关节
不动关节。其特点是通过纤维软骨来连接骨骼。

fibrous joints
Immoveable joints characterized by the presence of fibrocartilage connecting the bones.

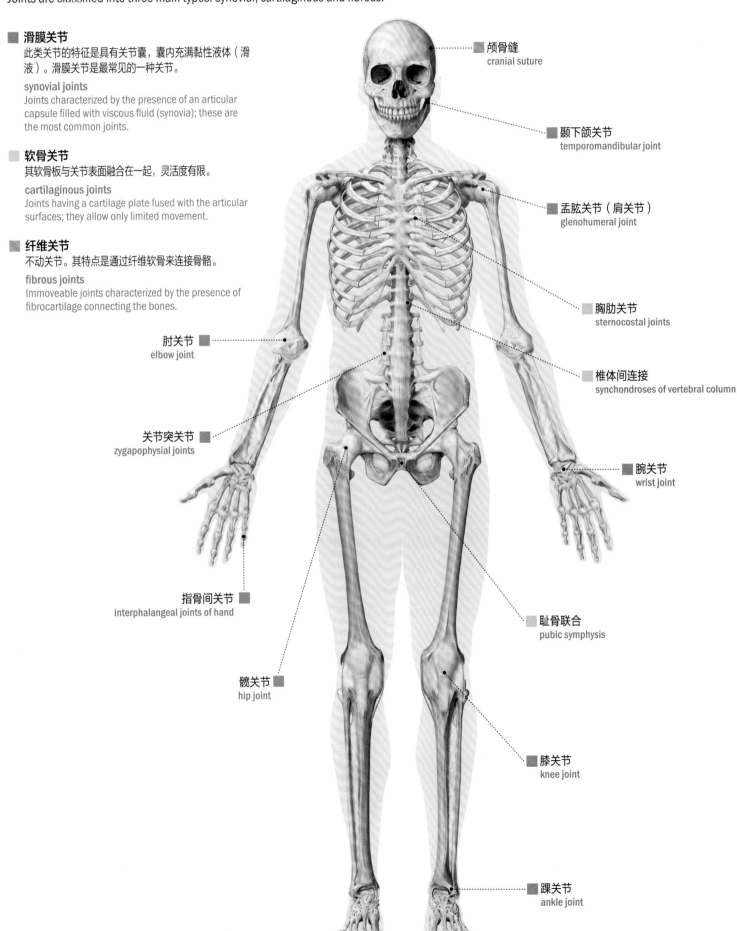

■ 颅骨缝
cranial suture

■ 颞下颌关节
temporomandibular joint

■ 盂肱关节（肩关节）
glenohumeral joint

■ 胸肋关节
sternocostal joints

■ 椎体间连接
synchondroses of vertebral column

■ 腕关节
wrist joint

■ 耻骨联合
pubic symphysis

■ 膝关节
knee joint

■ 踝关节
ankle joint

肘关节 ■
elbow joint

关节突关节 ■
zygapophysial joints

指骨间关节 ■
interphalangeal joints of hand

髋关节 ■
hip joint

编者注：椎骨与椎体

　　椎骨是构成脊柱的不规则骨。由前方短圆柱形的椎体和后方板状的椎弓组成。包括7块颈椎、12块胸椎、5块腰椎、5块骶椎和3~5块尾椎。幼年时为32块或33块，成年后骶、尾椎各融合成一块骶骨和尾骨，共26块。椎骨间由椎间盘和所属韧带构成具有特定生理弯曲的脊柱。

颅骨缝

纤维关节。连接两块颅骨并形成不规则的关节线，随着年龄增长，骨缝逐渐融合直至骨骼不再做任何移动。

cranial suture
Fibrous joint connecting two bones of the skull and forming an irregular line; the sutures fuse with age, preventing all movement of the bones.

颞下颌关节

滑膜关节。连接着下颌骨和颞骨，可使嘴开合。

temporomandibular joint
Synovial joint connecting the mandible with the temporal bone; it allows the mouth to open and close.

盂肱关节（肩关节）

滑膜关节。连接肱骨和肩胛骨，可使上臂沿三轴活动。

glenohumeral joint
Synovial joint connecting the humerus and the shoulder blade; it allows movements of the arm along three axes.

肘关节

滑膜关节。连接肱骨至桡骨和尺骨，可使前臂屈伸。

elbow joint
Synovial joint connecting the humerus to the radius and ulna; it allows mainly flexion and extension of the forearm.

胸肋关节

软骨关节。连接上七个肋软骨和胸骨。

sternocostal joints
Cartilaginous joints connecting the first seven costal cartilages to the sternum.

椎体间连接

软骨关节。通过椎间盘连接相邻两个椎骨。

synchondroses of vertebral column
Cartilaginous joints connecting the vertebral bodies of two adjacent vertebrae via an intervertebral disk.

关节突关节

滑膜关节。连接相邻两个椎骨关节突。

zygapophysial joints
Synovial joints connecting the articular apophyses of two adjacent vertebrae.

腕关节

滑膜关节。连接桡骨至舟状骨、半月骨和三角骨，可完成手部的活动。

wrist joint
Synovial joint connecting the radius to the scaphoid, semilunar and pyramidal bones; it allows movements of the hand.

指骨间关节

滑膜关节。连接两根指骨，使本节指骨的上部与下一节指骨的底部相连。可使手指屈伸。

interphalangeal joints of hand
Synovial joints connecting the upper part of a phalanx with the base of the next phalanx; they allow flexion and extension movements in the fingers.

耻骨联合

软骨关节。连接两块耻骨。

pubic symphysis
Cartilaginous joint connecting the two pubes.

膝关节

滑膜关节。连接股骨至胫骨和髌骨，可使小腿屈伸。

knee joint
Synovial joint connecting the femur to the tibia and patella; it allows mainly flexion and extension of the leg.

髋关节

滑膜关节。连接股骨头和髂骨，支撑身体重量，可使下肢完成多种动作。

hip joint
Synovial joint connecting the head of the femur to the iliac bone; it supports the body's weight and allows numerous movements of the lower limb.

踝关节

滑膜关节。连接胫骨、腓骨和距骨，可使足部屈伸。

ankle joint
Synovial joint connecting the tibia, fibula and talus; it allows flexion and extension of the foot.

软骨关节 | cartilaginous joints

软骨关节
关节的软骨板与关节表面融合在一起，灵活度有限。位于椎骨之间、耻骨之间和第一肋骨水平。

cartilaginous joints
Joints having a cartilage plate fused to articulating surfaces, allowing only limited movement; they are found between the vertebrae, pubic bones and at the level of the first rib.

椎体间连接
软骨关节。通过椎间盘连接相邻两个椎骨。

synchondroses of vertebral column
Cartilaginous joints connecting the vertebral bodies of two adjacent vertebrae via an intervertebral disk.

可左右移动 | From Left to Right
与其他椎骨不同，寰椎和枢椎之间并非由椎间盘相隔，而是由滑膜关节相连，从而可使头部旋转。

Unlike other vertebrae, the atlas and the axis are not separated by an intervertebral disk. Instead, they are connected by synovial joints that allow the head to rotate.

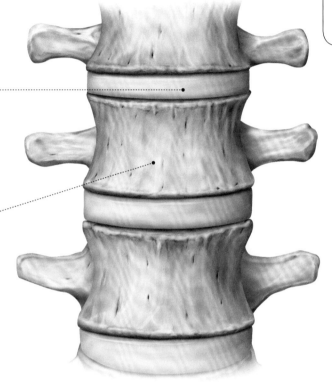

椎间盘
扁平圆形软骨结构。分隔相邻的两个椎骨，其弹性使得脊柱具有灵活性。

intervertebral disk
Flat, rounded cartilaginous structure separating two vertebrae; its elasticity provides mobility to the vertebral column.

椎体
厚圆盘状骨。组成椎骨前部。

vertebral body
Thick disk-shaped bony element comprising the anterior part of a vertebra.

椎间盘
扁平圆形软骨结构。分隔相邻两个椎骨，其弹性使得脊柱具有灵活性。

intervertebral disk
Flat, rounded cartilaginous structure separating two vertebrae; its elasticity provides mobility to the vertebral column.

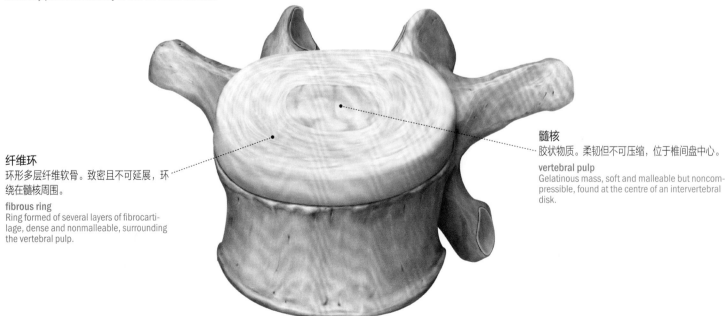

纤维环
环形多层纤维软骨。致密且不可延展，环绕在髓核周围。

fibrous ring
Ring formed of several layers of fibrocartilage, dense and nonmalleable, surrounding the vertebral pulp.

髓核
胶状物质。柔韧但不可压缩，位于椎间盘中心。

vertebral pulp
Gelatinous mass, soft and malleable but noncompressible, found at the centre of an intervertebral disk.

滑膜关节
此类关节的特征是具有关节囊，囊内充满黏性液体（滑液），遍布全身（包括肩、肘、腕、膝和踝）。

synovial joints
Joints characterized by the presence of an articulating capsule filled with a viscous liquid (synovia); they are found throughout the body (including the shoulder, elbow, wrist, knee and ankle).

滑膜关节横截面
cross section of a synovial joint

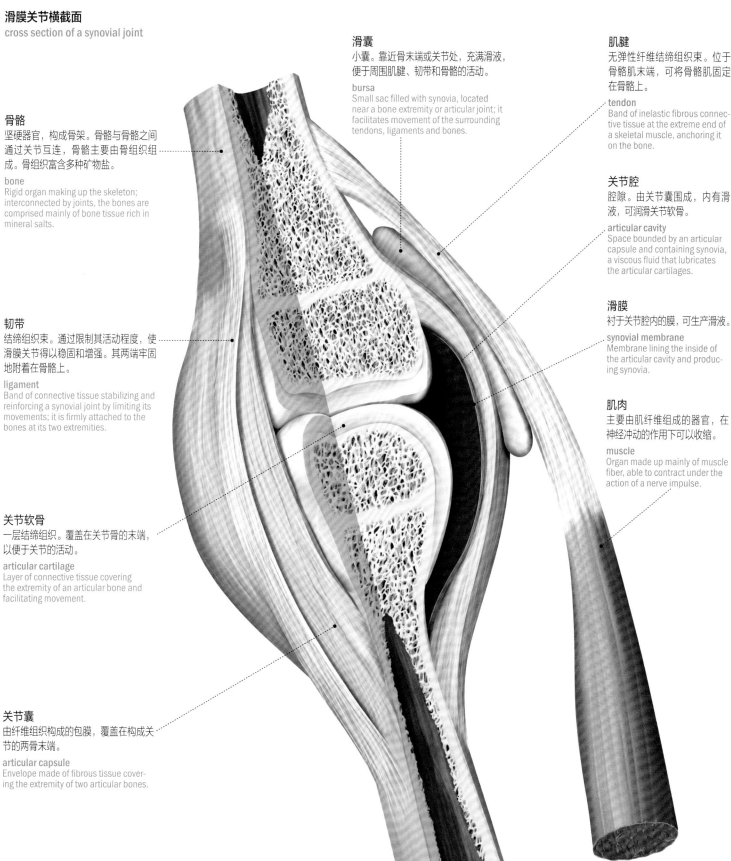

滑囊
小囊。靠近骨末端或关节处，充满滑液，便于周围肌腱、韧带和骨骼的活动。

bursa
Small sac filled with synovia, located near a bone extremity or articular joint; it facilitates movement of the surrounding tendons, ligaments and bones.

肌腱
无弹性纤维结缔组织束。位于骨骼肌末端，可将骨骼肌固定在骨骼上。

tendon
Band of inelastic fibrous connective tissue at the extreme end of a skeletal muscle, anchoring it on the bone.

骨骼
坚硬器官，构成骨架。骨骼与骨骼之间通过关节互连，骨骼主要由骨组织组成。骨组织富含多种矿物盐。

bone
Rigid organ making up the skeleton; interconnected by joints, the bones are comprised mainly of bone tissue rich in mineral salts.

关节腔
腔隙。由关节囊围成，内有滑液，可润滑关节软骨。

articular cavity
Space bounded by an articular capsule and containing synovia, a viscous fluid that lubricates the articular cartilages.

滑膜
衬于关节腔内的膜，可生产滑液。

synovial membrane
Membrane lining the inside of the articular cavity and producing synovia.

韧带
结缔组织束。通过限制其活动程度，使滑膜关节得以稳固和增强。其两端牢固地附着在骨骼上。

ligament
Band of connective tissue stabilizing and reinforcing a synovial joint by limiting its movements; it is firmly attached to the bones at its two extremities.

肌肉
主要由肌纤维组成的器官，在神经冲动的作用下可以收缩。

muscle
Organ made up mainly of muscle fiber, able to contract under the action of a nerve impulse.

关节软骨
一层结缔组织。覆盖在关节骨的末端，以便于关节的活动。

articular cartilage
Layer of connective tissue covering the extremity of an articular bone and facilitating movement.

关节囊
由纤维组织构成的包膜，覆盖在构成关节的两骨末端。

articular capsule
Envelope made of fibrous tissue covering the extremity of two articular bones.

滑膜关节图例
examples of synovial joints

髋关节前面观

髋关节:连接股骨头和髂骨的滑膜关节。它支撑体重并允许下肢各种活动。

hip: anterior view

Hip: synovial joint connecting the head of the femur to the iliac bone; it supports the body's weight and allows numerous movements of the lower limbs.

髋骨
hip bone

腹股沟韧带
inguinal ligament

关节囊
articular capsule

股骨
femur

踝侧面观

踝关节:连接胫骨、腓骨和距骨的滑膜关节。可使足部屈伸。

ankle: lateral view

Ankle: synovial joint connecting the tibia, fibula and talus; it allows flexion and extension of the foot.

各种各样的动作 | Variety of Movements

有些滑膜关节只允许做轻微的侧向活动,例如腕部骨骼;而有的关节可以沿着一个轴、两个轴甚至三个轴进行复杂的运动,例如肩关节。

Certain synovial joints allow only slight lateral movement (such as the bones of the carpus), while others allow complex movements along one, two, or even three axes (for example, the shoulder).

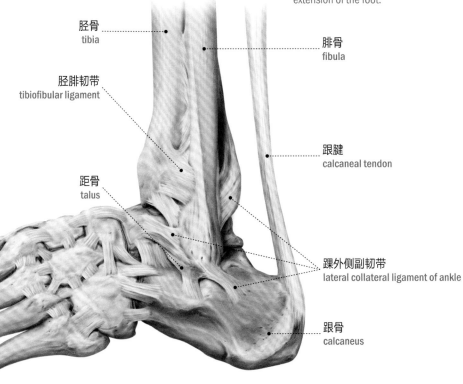

胫骨
tibia

腓骨
fibula

胫腓韧带
tibiofibular ligament

跟腱
calcaneal tendon

距骨
talus

踝外侧副韧带
lateral collateral ligament of ankle

跟骨
calcaneus

髋骨
成对骨。组成骨盆的最大部分。由儿时3块不同的骨骼（髂骨、耻骨和坐骨）融合而成。

iliac bone
Paired bone forming the largest part of the pelvis bone; it results from the fusion of three distinct bones in childhood; the ilium, the pubis and the ischium.

腹股沟韧带
连接两部分髂骨（髂骨和耻骨）的韧带。

inguinal ligament
Ligament connecting two parts of the iliac bone (ilium and pubis).

胫骨
大块的骨。构成小腿骨架内侧部分，在膝和踝关节之间。

tibia
Very large bone forming the inner part of the skeleton of the leg, between the knee and ankle joints.

胫腓韧带
连接胫骨和腓骨的下末端的韧带。

tibiofibular ligament
Ligament connecting the lower extremities of the tibia and fibula.

距骨
属于跗骨，位于跟骨上方，与胫骨和腓骨构成关节。

talus
Bone of the tarsus resting on the calcaneus and articulating with the tibia and fibula.

关节囊
由纤维组织构成的包膜。覆盖在髋关节骨的末端。

articular capsule
Envelope made of fibrous tissue covering the extremity of the articulated bones forming the hip joint.

股骨
成对的长骨。构成大腿骨架，位于髋关节和膝关节之间。

femur
Long paired bone forming the skeleton of the thigh, between the hip and knee joints.

腓骨
构成小腿骨架外侧部分的骨骼。在膝和踝关节之间。

fibula
Bone forming the outer part of the skeleton of the leg, between the knee and ankle joints.

跟腱
大肌腱。位于踝关节后侧，将小腿三头肌连至跟骨。

calcaneal tendon
Large tendon of the posterior face of the ankle, connecting the triceps surae to the calcaneus.

踝外侧副韧带
由三束纤维组成的韧带。分别将腓骨连接到胫骨、距骨及跟骨。

lateral collateral ligament of ankle
Ligament formed of three bunches of fibers connecting the fibula to the tibia, talus and calcaneus.

跟骨
属于跗骨，构成足跟部。跟腱和若干小腿肌肉附着其上。

calcaneus
Bone of the tarsus forming the heel of the foot and serving to attach the Achilles tendon and several calf muscles.

膝前面观

膝关节：连接股骨至胫骨和髌骨的滑膜关节。可使小腿屈伸。

knee: anterior view
Knee: synovial joint connecting the femur to the tibia and patella and allowing mainly flexion and extension of the leg.

股四头肌
四头肌。构成大腿的前部，叮使小腿伸展，大腿屈曲。

quadriceps muscle of thigh
Muscle having four heads forming the anterior part of the thigh; it allows extension of the leg and flexion of the thigh.

股骨
构成大腿骨架的骨骼。位于髋关节和膝关节之间。

femur
Bone forming the skeleton of the thigh, between the hip and knee joints.

髌骨
三角形骨。在膝部与股骨构成关节。

patella
Bone, triangular in shape, articulated with the femur at the knee.

关节囊
由纤维组织构成的包膜。覆盖在构成关节的两骨末端。

articular capsule
Envelope made of fibrous tissue covering the extremity of two articular bones.

髌腱
由髌骨延伸到胫骨的厚韧带。协助稳定膝关节。

patellar ligament
Thick ligament extending from the patella to the tibia; it assists in stabilizing the knee joint.

腓骨
构成小腿骨架外侧部分的骨骼。在膝和踝关节之间。

fibula
Bone forming the outer part of the skeleton of the leg, between the knee and ankle joints.

胫骨
大块的骨。构成小腿骨架内侧部分，在膝和踝关节之间。

tibia
Very large bone forming the inner part of the skeleton of the leg, between the knee and ankle joints.

膝扩展前面观

extended knee: anterior view

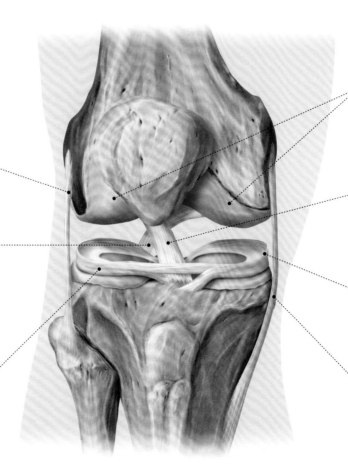

腓侧副韧带
位于膝关节外侧的韧带。连接股骨与腓骨，协助稳定膝关节。

fibular collateral ligament
Ligament extending from the femur to the fibula, on the external face of the knee, assisting in stabilizing its articulation.

后交叉韧带
位于膝关节内连接股骨和胫骨的韧带。限制胫骨的后移。

posterior cruciate ligament
Ligament located inside the articular capsule of the knee and connecting the femur to the tibia; it restrains backward movement of the tibia.

外侧半月板
位于膝关节外侧，并参与构成关节的半月形纤维软骨结构。

lateral meniscus
Semilunar fibrocartilaginous structure located on the outer side of the knee and assisting in its articulation.

股骨髁
股骨下端与胫骨构成关节的圆形突起。

condyles of femur
Rounded protrusions of the lower extremity of the femur, allowing articulation with the tibia.

前交叉韧带
位于膝关节内连接股骨和胫骨的韧带。限制胫骨的前移和旋转。

anterior cruciate ligament
Ligament located inside the articular capsule of the knee and connecting the femur to the tibia; it restrains forward movement of the tibia and its rotation.

内侧半月板
位于膝关节内侧，并参与构成关节的半月形纤维软骨结构。

medial meniscus
Semilunar fibrocartilaginous structure located on the inner side of the knee and assisting in its articulation.

胫侧副韧带
膝关节内侧连接股骨与胫骨的韧带。协助稳定膝关节。

tibial collateral ligament
Ligament extending from the femur to the tibia, on the internal face of the knee, assisting in stabilizing its articulation.

肩峰
肩胛骨的突起。与锁骨构成关节。

acromion
Bony protrusion of the shoulder
blade, articulating with the clavicle.

肩锁关节
滑膜关节。连接肩峰和锁骨。

acromioclavicular joint
Synovial joint connecting the
acromion and the clavicle.

肩前面观
肩关节：连接臂部和胸部的关节。包含两个
滑膜关节（盂肱关节和肩锁关节）。

shoulder: anterior view
Shoulder: joint connecting the arm with
the thorax, housing two synovial joints
(humeroscapular and acromioclavicular).

喙肩韧带
连接肩峰至肩胛骨喙突的韧带。

coracoacromial ligament
Ligament connecting the acromion to the
coracoid apophysis of the shoulder blade.

肩胛骨喙突
肩胛骨的突起。作为背部多个韧带和
肌肉的附着点。

coracoid process
Bony protrusion of the shoulder blade
serving to attach several ligaments and
muscles of the back.

锁骨
连接肩胛骨和胸骨的骨。

clavicle
Bone connecting the shoulder blade to the
sternum.

盂肱关节
滑膜关节。连接肱骨和肩胛骨，可使
上臂绕三轴活动。

glenohumeral joint
Synovial joint connecting the humerus
and the shoulder blade; it allows movements of the arm along three axes.

肩胛骨
三角形骨。位于胸廓后方，与锁骨和肱骨
相连，保护胸部，并作为背部多块肌肉的
止点。

scapula
Bone, triangular in shape, located behind the
thoracic cage, articulating with the clavicle
and humerus; it protects the thorax and
serves as the insertion point for several back
muscles.

肱骨
大块骨。位于肩和肘关节之间，构成上
臂骨架。

humerus
Very large bone making up the skeleton
of the arm, between the shoulder and
elbow joints.

各种动作 | Varied Movements

肩关节是全身最灵活的关节。可以屈伸、内收、外
展以及旋转。

The shoulder is the most mobile joint in the
body: it allows flexion and extension, adduction
and abduction, and rotation.

肘前面观
肘关节：滑膜关节。连接肱骨至桡骨和尺
骨，可使前臂旋转和屈伸。

elbow: anterior view
Elbow: synovial joint connecting the humerus to the radius and ulna, allowing
mainly rotation, flexion and extension
of the arm.

关节囊
由纤维组织构成的包膜。覆盖在构成关节的两
骨末端。

articular capsule
Envelope made of fibrous tissue covering the
extremity of two articular bones.

肱骨
大块骨。位于肩和肘关节之间，构成上臂
骨架。

humerus
Very large bone making up the skeleton of
the arm, between the shoulder and elbow
joints.

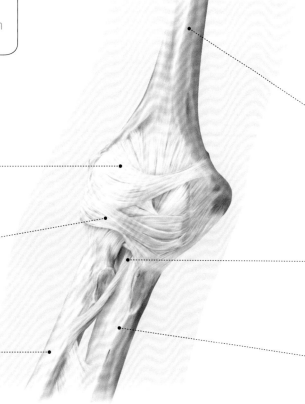

桡骨环状韧带
环绕桡骨头并将其固定在尺骨桡切迹的韧带。

annular ligament of radius
Ligament surrounding the head of the radius,
anchoring it in the radial notch of the ulna.

斜索
连接尺骨和桡骨的小韧带。

oblique cord
Small ligament connecting the ulna and radius.

桡骨
构成前臂骨架外侧部分的骨骼。在肘关节和腕
关节之间。

radius
Bone forming the outer part of the skeleton of the
forearm, between the elbow and wrist joints.

尺骨
构成前臂骨架内侧部分的骨骼。在肘关节和
腕关节之间。

ulna
Bone forming the inner part of the skeleton of the
forearm, between the elbow and wrist joints.

手腕和手背面观

腕部有多个连接桡骨、尺骨和腕骨
的关节，参与手的屈伸活动；手部
有许多关节，参与手指的活动。

wrist and hand: dorsal view

The wrist houses several joints
connecting the radius and ulna
to the carpal bones and allowing flexion and extension movements of the hand; the hand
houses various joints allowing
movements of the fingers.

桡骨
构成前臂骨架外侧部分的骨骼。
在肘关节和腕关节之间。

radius
Bone forming the outer part of
the skeleton of the forearm, between the elbow and wrist joints.

尺骨
构成前臂骨架内侧部分的骨骼。在肘关
节和腕关节之间。

ulna
Bone forming the inner part of the skeleton of the forearm, between the elbow
and wrist joints.

腕骨
构成腕关节的骨。

carpal bones
Bones making up the carpus.

掌指关节
滑膜关节。连接掌骨上部与近节指骨底
部，可使手指完成各种活动。

metacarpophalangeal joints
Synovial joints connecting the upper part of
the metacarpals to the base of the proximal
phalanges of the fingers; they allow various
movements of the fingers.

指间关节
滑膜关节。连接两根指骨，使本节指骨的上部与
下一节指骨的底部相连。可使手指屈伸。

interphalangeal joints of hand
Synovial joints connecting the upper part of a phalanx with the base of the next phalanx; they allow
flexion and extension movements in the fingers.

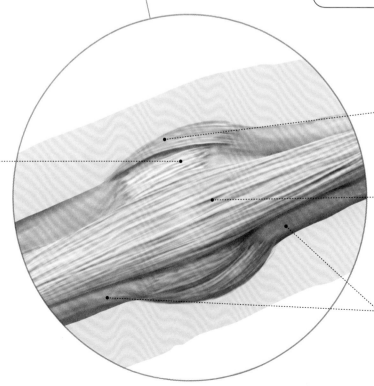

精确工具 | A Precise Tool

手腕和手包含大约20个关节，可做出如抓取物
品等多种精细动作。
The wrist and hand contain some 20 joints
that allow for very detailed mobility for,
among other things, gripping objects.

侧副韧带
连接两指骨的韧带。协助稳定相应的指
间关节。

collateral ligament
Ligament connecting two phalanges of
a finger, assisting in stabilizing the corresponding interphalangeal joint.

肌腱
无弹性纤维结缔组织束。连接指骨到手
部和前臂的肌肉。

tendon
Band of inelastic fibrous connective
tissue, connecting the phalanges to the
muscles of the hand and forearm.

关节囊
由纤维组织构成的包膜。覆盖在构成关
节的两骨末端。

articular capsule
Envelope made of fibrous tissue covering the extremity of two articular bones.

指骨
组成手指的骨。除了拇指有两个指骨，
其余每个手指有三个指骨。

phalanges of fingers
Bones forming the skeleton of the
fingers. Each finger has three phalanges,
except the thumb that has two.

胸椎侧面观
胸部的12块胸椎。由椎骨关节突关节互连。

thoracic vertebrae: lateral view
The 12_thoracic vertebrae, located at the thorax, are interconnected by zygapophysial joints.

横突
骨性突起。位于椎骨侧面，作为韧带的附着点。

transverse process
Bony protrusion on the side of a vertebra serving to attach ligaments.

棘上韧带
长韧带。连接椎骨棘突。

supraspinous ligament
Long ligament connecting the spinous apophyses of the vertebrae.

椎间孔
两块相邻椎骨之间的孔。可使脊神经通过。

intervertebral foramen
Aperture between two adjacent vertebrae, allowing especially for the passage of a spinal nerve.

棘突
骨性突起。位于椎骨后部，作为背部肌肉和韧带的附着点。

spinous process
Bony protrusion behind a vertebra serving to attach the muscles and ligaments of the back.

关节突关节
滑膜关节。连接相邻两块椎骨关节突。

zygapophysial joints
Synovial joints connecting the articular apophyses of two adjacent vertebrae.

横突间韧带
连接相邻两块椎骨横突的韧带。

intertransverse ligament
Ligament connecting the transverse apophyses of two adjacent vertebrae.

椎体
厚圆盘状骨。组成椎骨前部。

vertebral body
Thick disk-shaped bony element comprising the anterior part of a vertebra.

关节突
骨性突起。位于椎弓根上，可使相邻椎骨形成关节。

articular process
Bony protrusion on the neural arch of a vertebra, allowing its articulation with adjacent vertebrae.

前纵韧带
长韧带。覆盖脊柱前部，从颅底一直到骶骨。

anterior longitudinal ligament
Long ligament covering the anterior face of the vertebral column, from the base of the skull to the sacrum.

棘间韧带
连接相邻两块椎骨棘突的韧带。

interspinous ligament
Ligament connecting the spinous apophyses of two adjacent vertebrae.

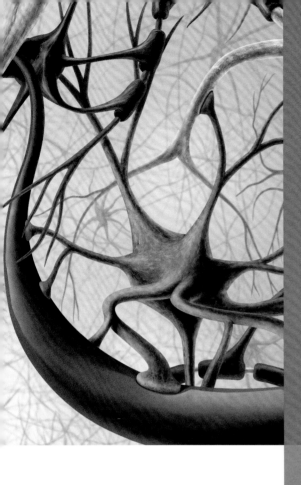

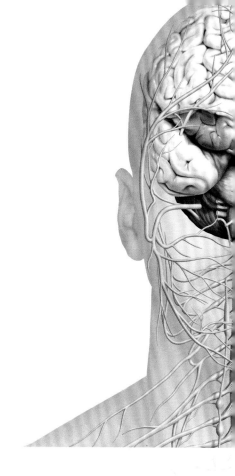

神经系统 Nervous system

神经系统由包括大脑、脊髓和神经在内的多个结构组成，实现人体的感觉功能、运动功能、自主功能以及思想功能。更具体地说，神经系统控制着人体的脏器功能，协调各种动作，于身体各部分之间传递感觉信息和运动信息，调控情绪等等。神经系统的功能主要通过神经元来实现。神经元是一类特殊的细胞，彼此之间通过电信号和化学信号进行交流。

The nervous system is a group of structures (brain, spinal cord, nerves) that fulfill the body's sensory, motor, autonomous, and mental functions. More specifically, it controls organ function, coordinates movements, transmits sensory and motor information between various parts of the body, regulates the emotions, etc. The nervous system operates mainly through neurons, specialised cells that communicate with each other using electrical and chemical signals.

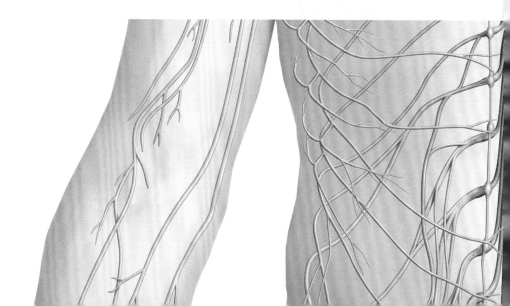

神经系统的组成

神经系统由两个独立部分组成并各有分工：中枢神经系统和周围神经系统。

structure of nervous system

The nervous system is made up of two distinct entities with defined roles: the central nervous system and the peripheral nervous system.

■ 脑

中枢神经系统的一部分。由颅骨包裹，包括大脑、小脑和脑干。负责感官知觉、大部分动作、记忆、语言、反射和各种生命功能。

brain

Part of the central nervous system enclosed in the skull, consisting of the brain, cerebellum and brain stem; it is responsible for sensory perception, most movements, memory, language, reflexes and vital functions.

■ 脊髓

中枢神经系统的一部分。位于脊柱内，在脊神经和脑之间传递神经信息。

spinal cord

Part of the central nervous system located in the vertebral column; it transmits nerve information between the spinal nerves and encephalon, and conversely.

■ 脑神经

12对脑神经。从脑干发出，为头部和颈部提供神经感知，并具有运动或感觉功能。

cranial nerves

Group of 12_pairs of nerves emerging from the brain stem, providing nerve sensation to the head and neck and serving a motor or sensory function.

■ 脊神经

31对混合神经。包括感觉神经和运动神经，从脊髓发出，提供除面部以外身体所有部分的神经感知。

spinal nerves

Group of 31_pairs of mixed (sensory and motor) nerves emerging from the spinal cord, providing nerve sensations to all parts of the body, except the face.

■ 中枢神经系统

神经系统的一部分。由大脑和脊髓构成，中枢神经系统负责解析感觉信息并发出动作指令。

central nervous system

Part of the nervous system formed by the brain and the spinal cord that interprets sensory information and initiates motor commands.

■ 周围神经系统

神经系统的一部分。由脑神经和脊神经组成，把感受器的感觉信息传送到中枢神经系统，并把中枢神经系统的运动指令传送到肌肉和腺体。

peripheral nervous system

Part of the nervous system made up of cranial and spinal nerves, carrying messages from sensory receptors to the central nervous system and transmitting motor commands from the central nervous system to the muscles and glands.

长短不一 | Variable Length

每个神经元都有一个突起状的结构，称为轴突。轴突的长度短则1毫米，长则达1米以上。

Each neuron has an extension, called an axon, that may measure between 1mm and more than 1m in length.

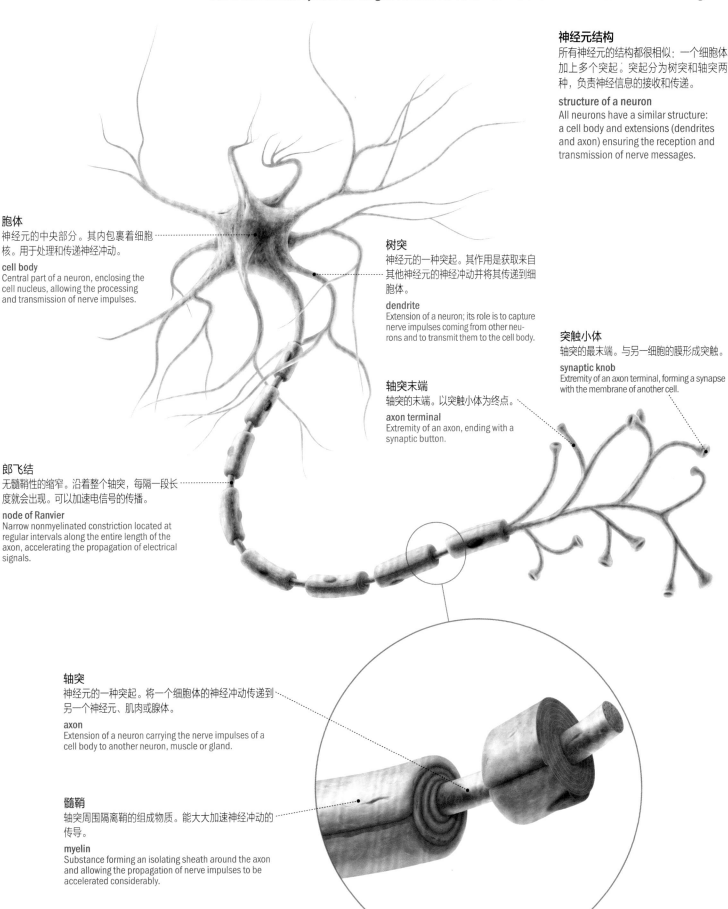

神经元
神经系统的细胞。以电信号和化学信号的形式传递信息。

neuron
Cell of the nervous system allowing information to be carried in the form of electrical and chemical signals.

神经元结构
所有神经元的结构都很相似：一个细胞体加上多个突起。突起分为树突和轴突两种，负责神经信息的接收和传递。

structure of a neuron
All neurons have a similar structure: a cell body and extensions (dendrites and axon) ensuring the reception and transmission of nerve messages.

胞体
神经元的中央部分。其内包裹着细胞核。用于处理和传递神经冲动。

cell body
Central part of a neuron, enclosing the cell nucleus, allowing the processing and transmission of nerve impulses.

树突
神经元的一种突起。其作用是获取来自其他神经元的神经冲动并将其传递到细胞体。

dendrite
Extension of a neuron; its role is to capture nerve impulses coming from other neurons and to transmit them to the cell body.

突触小体
轴突的最末端。与另一细胞的膜形成突触。

synaptic knob
Extremity of an axon terminal, forming a synapse with the membrane of another cell.

轴突末端
轴突的末端。以突触小体为终点。

axon terminal
Extremity of an axon, ending with a synaptic button.

郎飞结
无髓鞘性的缩窄。沿着整个轴突，每隔一段长度就会出现。可以加速电信号的传播。

node of Ranvier
Narrow nonmyelinated constriction located at regular intervals along the entire length of the axon, accelerating the propagation of electrical signals.

轴突
神经元的一种突起。将一个细胞体的神经冲动传递到另一个神经元、肌肉或腺体。

axon
Extension of a neuron carrying the nerve impulses of a cell body to another neuron, muscle or gland.

髓鞘
轴突周围隔离鞘的组成物质。能大大加速神经冲动的传导。

myelin
Substance forming an isolating sheath around the axon and allowing the propagation of nerve impulses to be accelerated considerably.

神经冲动 | nerve impulse

神经冲动
电信号。沿轴突传递，在身体各部位传递运动或感觉信息。

nerve impulse
Electrical signal running along an axon and allowing motor or sensory messages to be transmitted between different areas of the body.

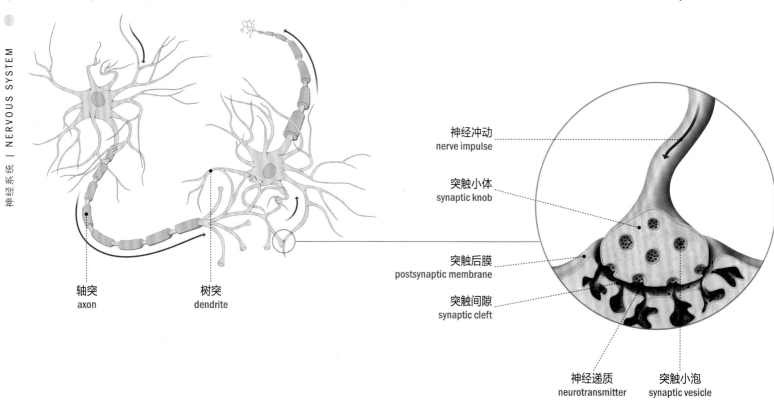

神经冲动
nerve impulse

突触小体
synaptic knob

突触后膜
postsynaptic membrane

突触间隙
synaptic cleft

神经递质
neurotransmitter

突触小泡
synaptic vesicle

轴突
axon

树突
dendrite

神经组织 | nervous tissue

神经组织
由紧密缠绕在一起的神经元和支持细胞构成的组织。构成神经系统的各种结构（脑、脊髓、神经节和神经）。

nervous tissue
Tissue made up of closely intertwined neurons and support cells, forming the structures of the nervous system (brain, spinal cord, nerve ganglions, and nerves).

中枢神经系统组织
central nervous system tissue

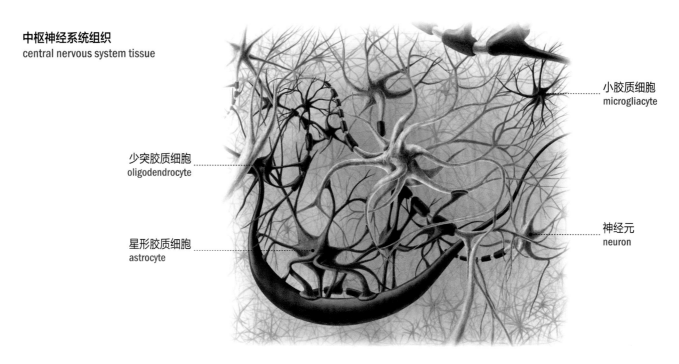

少突胶质细胞
oligodendrocyte

星形胶质细胞
astrocyte

小胶质细胞
microgliacyte

神经元
neuron

轴突

神经元的一种突起。将一个细胞体的神经冲动传递到另一个神经元、肌肉或腺体。

axon

Extension of a neuron carrying the nerve impulses of a cell body to another neuron, muscle or gland.

树突

神经元的一种突起。其作用是获取来自其他神经元的神经冲动并将其传递到细胞体。

dendrite

Extension of a neuron; its role is to capture nerve impulses coming from other neurons and to transmit them to the cell body.

突触

神经元与另一个细胞（神经元、肌肉纤维以及腺体的分泌细胞）之间的接触区。确保信息的传递。

synapse

Contact zone between a neuron and another cell (neuron, muscle fiber, secretory cell of a gland), ensuring the transmission of messages.

神经冲动

电信号。沿轴突传递，在身体各部位传递运动或感觉信息。

nerve impulse

Electrical signal running along an axon and allowing motor or sensory messages to be transmitted between different areas of the body.

突触小体

轴突的最末端。与另一细胞的膜形成突触。

synaptic knob

Extremity of an axon terminal, forming a synapse with the membrane of another cell.

神经递质

化学物质。由神经元在突触处释放，可实现两个神经元之间的信息传递。

neurotransmitter

Chemical substance released by a neuron at a synapse, allowing transmission of a message to another cell.

突触后膜

突触的细胞膜。膜上有许多受体，专供与神经递质连接。

postsynaptic membrane

Cell membrane of a synapse, having numerous receptors onto which neurotransmitters specifically attach.

突触间隙

突触的狭小空隙。神经递质在此释放。

synaptic cleft

Thin space at a synapse, in which neurotransmitters are released.

突触小泡

液泡。位于轴突的最末端，内含神经递质。

synaptic vesicle

Vacuole located in the axon terminal and containing neurotransmitters.

少突胶质细胞

构成中枢神经系统的轴突髓鞘的细胞。

oligodendrocyte

Cell forming the myelin sheath of axons of the central nervous system.

星形胶质细胞

具有多个突起的细胞。为中枢神经系统的神经元提供支撑、营养和保护。

astrocyte

Cell having multiple extensions, ensuring support, nutrition and protection of the neurons of the central nervous system.

小胶质细胞

免疫细胞。可消灭异物（感染性病原体）和吞噬死亡的神经组织细胞。

microgliacyte

Cell of the immune system, destroying foreign bodies (infectious agents) and the dead cells of nerve tissue.

神经元

神经系统的细胞。以电信号和化学信号的形式传递信息。

neuron

Cell of the nervous system allowing information to be carried in the form of electrical and chemical signals.

神经系统 | NERVOUS SYSTEM

中枢神经系统

神经系统的一部分，由脑和脊髓构成。中枢神经系统负责解析感觉信息并发出动作指令。

central nervous system

Part of the nervous system formed by the brain and the spinal cord that interprets sensory information and initiates motor commands.

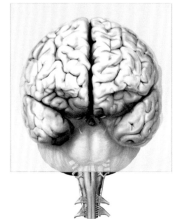

脑

中枢神经系统的一部分，由颅骨包裹。包括大脑、小脑和脑干。负责感官知觉、大部分运动、记忆、语言、反射以及其他生命功能。

brain

Part of the central nervous system enclosed in the skull, consisting of the brain, cerebellum and brain stem; it is responsible for sensory perception, most movements, memory, language, reflexes and vital functions.

脑冠状面
frontal section of brain

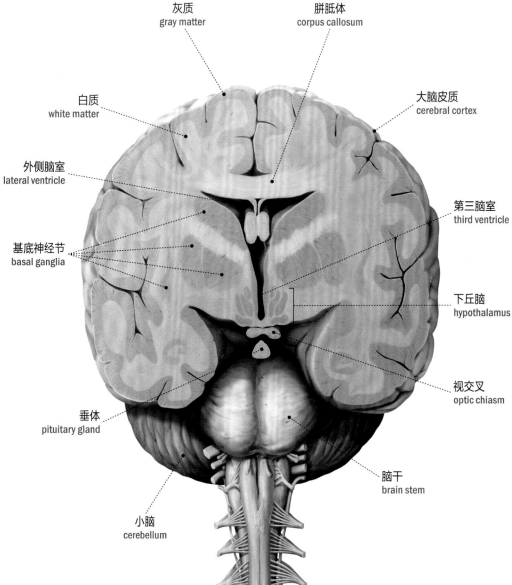

灰质
gray matter

胼胝体
corpus callosum

白质
white matter

大脑皮质
cerebral cortex

外侧脑室
lateral ventricle

第三脑室
third ventricle

基底神经节
basal ganglia

下丘脑
hypothalamus

垂体
pituitary gland

视交叉
optic chiasm

脑干
brain stem

小脑
cerebellum

速度很快 | Speed with a Capital S

当轴突有髓鞘包裹时，神经冲动的传递速度会加快，可达150米/秒。

Neural impulses may travel as fast as 150m/s when the axon is covered with a myelin sheath.

灰质
中枢神经系统物质。由神经元的细胞体构成，确保神经冲动的处理。

gray matter
Substance of the central nervous system formed by the cell bodies of neurons; it ensures the processing of nerve impulses.

胼胝体
白质带。连接大脑的两个半球。

corpus callosum
Band of white matter connecting the two cerebral hemispheres.

白质
中枢神经系统物质。由神经元的突起组成，连接脑和脊髓的各部分。

white matter
Substance of the central nervous system formed by extensions of the neurons; it connects various parts of the encephalon and spinal cord.

大脑皮质
大脑的浅层。由灰质组成，负责最高级别的神经功能。

cerebral cortex
Superficial layer of the cerebrum, made up of gray matter, assuring the most advanced nerve functions.

外侧脑室
大脑第三脑室两侧的两个腔。协助产生脑脊液。

lateral ventricle
Each of the two cavities located on either side of the third ventricle of the cerebrum, assisting in the production of cephalorachidian fluid.

第三脑室
脑腔。协助产生脑脊液。

third ventricle
Cavity of the encephalon assisting in the production of cephalorachidian fluid.

基底神经节
由灰质构成的核团。位于大脑中央，控制运动的精准度，并在学习复杂运动的过程中发挥一定作用。

basal ganglia
Formations of gray matter located in the central part of the cerebrum, controlling the precision of movements and playing a role in the learning of complex movements.

下丘脑
由灰质构成的一堆小核团。调节垂体的激素分泌，控制自主神经系统的活动。

hypothalamus
All the small formations of gray matter, controlling the hormonal secretions of the pituitary gland and the activity of the autonomic nervous system.

垂体
内分泌腺。由下丘脑控制，能分泌九种主要激素。这些激素尤在生长、泌乳、血压和尿量调节等方面发挥作用。

pituitary gland
Endocrine gland that is controlled by the hypothalamus and that secretes nine major hormones that act especially on growth, lactation, blood pressure and urine retention.

视交叉
由双眼视神经的接合部形成的结构。两眼的神经纤维有部分相交。

optic chiasm
Structures formed by the juncture of the optic nerves of the right and left eyes, whose fibers partially intersect.

脑干
脑的一部分。位于脊髓的延伸处，调节许多重要机能并确保脊髓、大脑和小脑之间的信息传输。

brain stem
Part of the encephalon located in the extension of the spinal cord, regulating numerous vital functions and ensuring transmissions between the spinal cord, cerebrum and cerebellum.

小脑
脑的一部分。主要控制运动协调、平衡、肌肉张力和姿态。

cerebellum
Part of the encephalon, controlling mainly motor coordination, balance, muscle tone and posture.

大脑上面观

大脑：脑的最大和最复杂的部分。含有高级神经功能（包括运动和语言活动）的控制中心。

cerebrum: superior view

Cerebrum: largest and most complex part of the encephalon, containing the control center of upper nerve functions (including motor activities and language).

左半球
大脑的左半部分。控制身体右侧的运动。擅长分析和逻辑思维。

left hemisphere
Left part of the cerebrum, controlling the movements of the right side of the body; it also specializes in analysis and logical thinking.

右半球
大脑的右半部分。控制身体左侧的运动。与艺术和形象思维相关。

right hemisphere
Right part of the cerebrum, controlling the movements of the left side of the body; it is involved in artistic activities.

脑回
大脑半球的表面部分。被脑沟分隔。

gyri
Portions of the surface of a cerebral hemisphere bounded by a sulcus.

纵裂
分隔大脑两个半球的深脊。

longitudinal fissure
Deep ridge separating the two cerebral hemispheres.

脑沟
大脑两个脑回之间的凹陷。

sulci
Depressions surrounding two convolutions of the cerebrum.

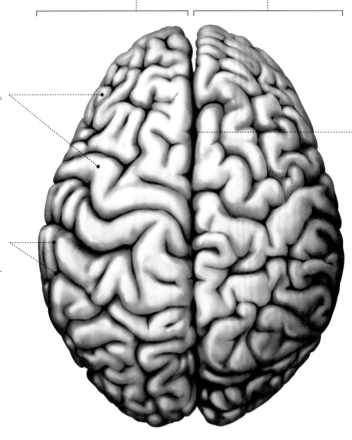

大脑外侧观
cerebrum: lateral view

顶叶
位于大脑中部的脑叶。参与味觉、触觉、疼痛和理解语言。

parietal lobe
Lobe located in the middle part of the cerebrum, involved in taste, touch, pain and language comprehension.

额叶
位于大脑前部，前额后方的脑叶。负责推理、计划、自主运动、情感和言语表达。

frontal lobe
Lobe located in the anterior part of the cerebrum, behind the forehead, responsible for reasoning, planning, voluntary movements, emotions and spoken language.

枕叶
位于大脑后部的脑叶。负责视觉。

occipital lobe
Lobe located at the back of the cerebrum, playing a role in vision.

颞叶
位于大脑外侧的脑叶。负责听力和记忆。

temporal lobe
Lobe located in the lateral part of the cerebrum, responsible for hearing and memory.

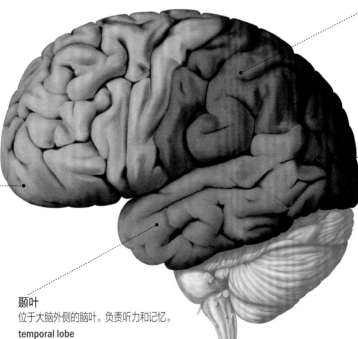

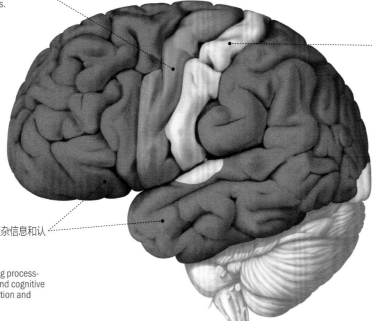

大脑皮质
大脑的浅层。由灰质组成，负责最高级别的神经功能。

cerebral cortex
Superficial layer of the cerebrum, made up of gray matter, assuring the most advanced nerve functions.

运动皮质
大脑的一部分。调节自主运动。

motor cortex
Part of the cerebrum regulating voluntary movements.

感觉皮质
大脑的一部分。构成感知的基础。

sensory cortex
Part of the cerebrum forming the basis of perceptions.

联合皮质
大脑的一部分。负责处理复杂信息和认知功能，如记忆和语言。

association cortex
Part of the cerebrum ensuring processing of complex information and cognitive functions, such as memorization and language.

液体保护 | Liquid Protection

中枢神经系统的各个器官被一种由脑室产生的液体所包围，即脑脊液。脑脊液由水、蛋白质和营养成分组成，起到减震作用。

The organs of the central nervous system are surrounded with a liquid produced by the cerebral ventricles: cephalorachidian liquid. Composed of water, protein, and nutrients, it acts as a shock_absorber.

边缘系统
与情绪、记忆和学习相关的神经结构。

limbic system
All the nerve structures involved in emotions, memory and learning.

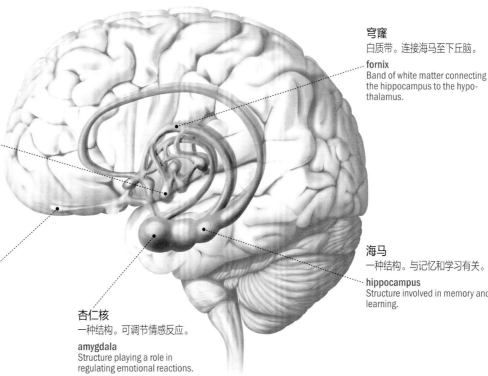

穹窿
白质带。连接海马至下丘脑。

fornix
Band of white matter connecting the hippocampus to the hypothalamus.

下丘脑
由灰质组成的小核团。调节垂体的激素分泌，控制自主神经系统活动。

hypothalamus
All the small formations of gray matter, controlling the hormonal secretions of the pituitary gland and the activity of the autonomic nervous system.

嗅球
膨大的神经组织。连接嗅觉神经，起中继作用，把嗅觉信息传递到大脑。

olfactory bulb
Enlargement of nerve tissue connected to the olfactory nerves; it serves as a relay in transmitting olfactory information to the cerebrum.

杏仁核
一种结构。可调节情感反应。

amygdala
Structure playing a role in regulating emotional reactions.

海马
一种结构。与记忆和学习有关。

hippocampus
Structure involved in memory and learning.

小脑截面
小脑：脑的一部分。主要控制运动协调、身体平衡、肌肉张力和身体姿态。

section of cerebellum
Cerebellum: part of the encephalon controlling mainly motor coordination, balance, muscle tone and posture.

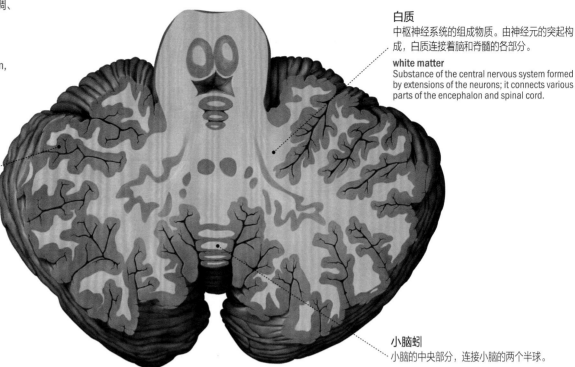

白质
中枢神经系统的组成物质。由神经元的突起构成，白质连接着脑和脊髓的各部分。

white matter
Substance of the central nervous system formed by extensions of the neurons; it connects various parts of the encephalon and spinal cord.

灰质
中枢神经系统的组成物质。由神经元的细胞体构成，灰质是突触的聚集所在，负责神经冲动的处理。

gray matter
Substance of the central nervous system formed by the cell bodies of neurons; home to the synapses, it ensures the processing of nerve impulses.

小脑蚓
小脑的中央部分，连接小脑的两个半球。

vermis
Central part of the cerebellum, uniting the two cerebellar hemispheres.

小脑半球体
小脑两个对称半球的一个。

cerebellar hemisphere
Each of the two symmetrical halves of the cerebellum.

脑干后外侧观
脑干：脑的一部分。位于脊髓的延伸部，调节许多重要功能，确保脊髓、大脑和小脑之间信息的传输。

brain stem: posterolateral view
Brain stem: part of the encephalon located in the extension of the spinal cord, regulating numerous vital functions and ensuring transmissions between the spinal cord, brain and cerebellum.

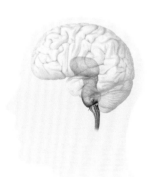

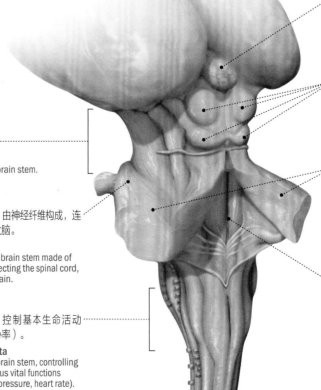

松果体
大脑的内分泌腺。可分泌褪黑素，影响精子形成或月经周期。

pineal gland
Endocrine gland of the brain secreting melatonin and influencing the formation of spermatozoa or the menstrual cycle.

丘
中脑背侧面上的膨出。有视觉和听觉功能。

colliculi
Enlargements on the dorsal face of the midbrain, playing a role in vision and hearing.

小脑脚
成束的白质。连接小脑和脑干的特定部位。

cerebellar peduncles
Bundles of white matter connecting the cerebellum to certain parts of the brain stem.

第四脑室
小脑和脑干之间的空腔。协助产生脑脊液。

fourth ventricle
Cavity between the cerebellum and brain stem, assisting in the production of cephalorachidian fluid.

中脑
脑干的上部。

midbrain
Upper part of the brain stem.

脑桥
脑干的中央部分。由神经纤维构成，连接脊髓，小脑和大脑。

pons
Central part of the brain stem made of nerve fibers, connecting the spinal cord, cerebellum and brain.

延髓
脑干的下部分。控制基本生命活动（呼吸、血压、心率）。

medulla oblongata
Lower part of the brain stem, controlling especially numerous vital functions (breathing, blood pressure, heart rate).

脑膜
膜状结构。包裹和保护脊髓和脑。

meninges
Membranes enveloping and protecting the spinal cord and encephalon.

帽状腱膜
覆盖颅骨的纤维层。位于额肌和枕肌之间。

epicranial aponeurosis
Fibrous layer covering the skull, between the frontal and occipital muscles.

头皮
头颅上的皮肤。上覆头发。

scalp
Part of the skin of the head covered with hair.

颅骨
骨骼结构。由八块骨骼组成（四块规则形状和四块不规则形状），覆盖并保护着脑。

skull
Bony structure formed of eight bones (four even bones and four odd bones) covering and protecting the brain.

大脑皮质
大脑浅层。由灰质组成，负责最高级别的神经功能。

cerebral cortex
Superficial layer of the cerebrum, made up of gray matter, assuring the most advanced nerve functions.

硬脑膜
外层脑膜。厚且坚韧，由两层纤维组织构成。

dura mater
Outer meninx, thick and resistant, formed of two sheets of fibrous tissue.

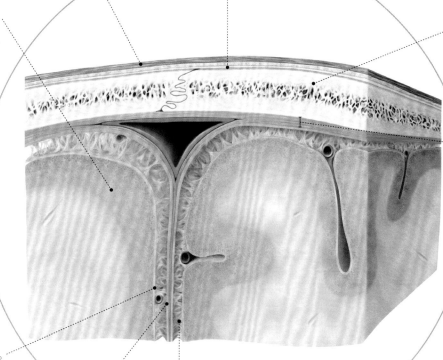

软脑膜
内层脑膜。紧贴于脑和脊髓。

pia mater
Inner meninx, narrowly covering the brain and spinal cord.

蛛网膜
中间脑膜。与硬脑膜相连，并通过蛛网膜下腔与软脑膜分离。

arachnoid
Middle meninx, attached to the dura mater and separated from the pia mater by the subarachnoid space.

蛛网膜下腔
在蛛网膜和软脑膜之间的腔隙。含有脑脊液和脑的主要血管。

subarachnoid space
Space between the arachnoid and pia mater, containing cephalorachidian fluid and the main blood vessels of the encephalon.

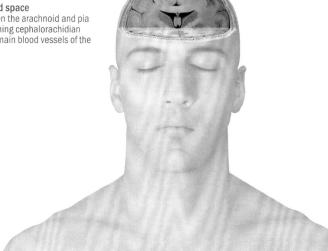

富含神经元 | Rich in Neurons

尽管小脑质量只占脑的10%，却包含了脑神经元总数的一半之多。

The cerebellum contains half of the neurons in the brain, even though it represents only 10% of the brain's total mass.

脊髓

中枢神经系统的一部分。位于脊柱内，负责将神经信息在脊神经和脑之间来回传送。

spinal cord

Part of the central nervous system located in the vertebral column, transmitting nerve information from the spinal nerves to the brain and back.

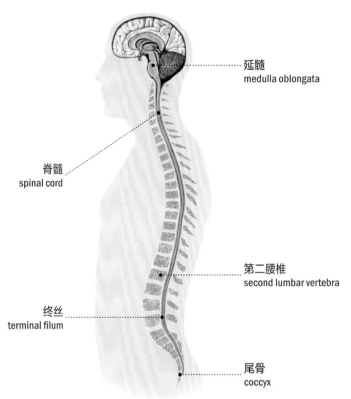

延髓
medulla oblongata

脊髓
spinal cord

第二腰椎
second lumbar vertebra

终丝
terminal filum

尾骨
coccyx

脊柱横截面

脊柱：由33个椎骨组成。从颅骨延伸至骨盆，支撑头部及躯干，内部包含脊髓。

cross section of the vertebral column

Vertebral column: bony grouping of 33 vertebrae, extending from the skull to the pelvis; it supports the head and trunk and contains the spinal cord.

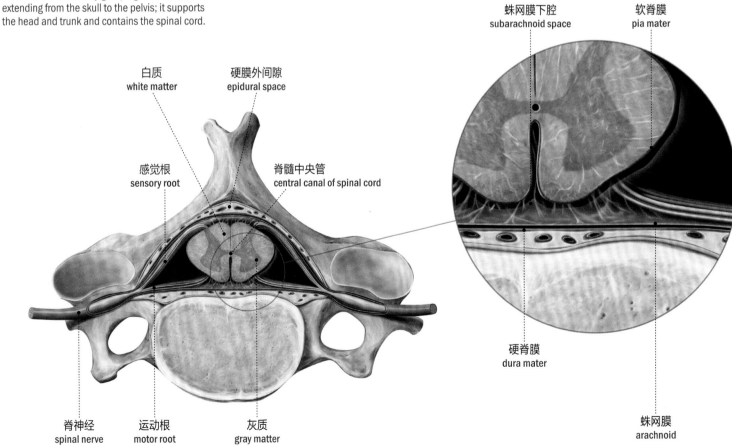

白质
white matter

硬膜外间隙
epidural space

感觉根
sensory root

脊髓中央管
central canal of spinal cord

脊神经
spinal nerve

运动根
motor root

灰质
gray matter

蛛网膜下腔
subarachnoid space

软脊膜
pia mater

硬脊膜
dura mater

蛛网膜
arachnoid

脊髓
中枢神经系统的一部分。位于延髓和第二腰椎之间的脊柱内。

spinal cord
Part of the central nervous system located in the vertebral column, between the medulla oblongata and the second lumbar vertebra.

终丝
软脊膜的纤维延伸。从脊髓的末端延伸到尾骨。

terminal filum
Fibrous extension of the pia mater, extending from the extremity of the spinal cord to the coccyx.

白质
中枢神经系统的一部分。由神经纤维构成，连接脑和脊髓的各个部分。

white matter
Substance of the central nervous system formed by extensions of the neurons; it connects various parts of the encephalon and spinal cord.

硬膜外间隙
硬脊膜和椎骨之间的空腔。腔内充满脂肪组织和血管，保护脊髓不受损伤。

epidural space
Cavity between the dura mater and the vertebrae, filled with adipose tissue and blood vessels; it protects the spinal cord from trauma.

感觉根
脊神经的分支，将感觉信息从身体感觉末梢神经传送到脊髓。

sensory root
Branch of a spinal nerve transmitting sensory information from the periphery of the body to the spinal cord.

脊髓中央管
位于脊髓中心的管道。与第四脑室相连并输送脑脊液。

central canal of spinal cord
Canal located at the center of the spinal cord, communicating with the fourth cerebral ventricle and transporting cephalorachidian fluid.

脊神经
来自于脊髓的混合神经。支配除了面部以外的身体所有部分。

spinal nerve
Each of the mixed nerves emerging from the spinal cord and innervating all parts of the body, except the face.

运动根
脊神经的分支，将运动信息从脊髓传送到外周，特别是肌肉组织。

motor root
Branch of a spinal nerve transmitting motor information from the spinal cord to the periphery of the body, especially the muscles.

灰质
由神经元细胞体构成的中枢神经物质，确保了神经冲动的处理。

gray matter
Substance of the central nervous system formed by the cell bodies of neurons; it ensures the processing of nerve impulses.

延髓
脑干的下部分。控制基本生命活动（呼吸、血压、心率）。

medulla oblongata
Lower part of the brain stem, controlling especially numerous vital functions (breathing, blood pressure, heart rate).

第二腰椎
位于第一腰椎和第三腰椎之间的椎体。

second lumbar vertebra
Vertebra located between the first and third lumbar vertebrae.

尾骨
小三角骨。由四块尾椎骨于成年期之初融合而成，构成脊柱的下末端。

coccyx
Small triangular bone formed by the fusion, at the start of adulthood, of the four coccygeal vertebrae, and making up the lower extremity of the vertebral column.

蛛网膜下腔
蛛网膜和软脊膜之间的腔隙，含有脑脊液和血管。

subarachnoid space
Space between the arachnoid and pia mater, containing cephalorachidian fluid and blood vessels.

软脊膜
内层脑膜。紧贴于脑和脊髓。

pia mater
Inner meninx, narrowly covering the brain and spinal cord.

硬脊膜
外层脑膜。厚且坚韧，由两层纤维组织组成。

dura mater
Outer meninx, thick and resistant, formed of two sheets of fibrous tissue.

蛛网膜
中间脑膜。与硬脑膜相连，通过蛛网膜下腔与软脑膜相隔。

arachnoid
Middle meninx, attached to the dura mater and separated from the pia mater by the subarachnoid space.

周围神经系统

神经系统的一部分。由脑神经和脊神经组成，把感受器的感觉信息传送到中枢神经系统，并把中枢神经系统的运动指令传送到肌肉和腺体。

peripheral nervous system
Part of the nervous system made up of cranial and spinal nerves, carrying messages from sensory receptors to the central nervous system and transmitting motor commands from the central nervous system to the muscles and glands.

混合神经截面

混合神经：由神经纤维组成的长索。在中枢神经系统和身体其他部分之间传递感觉和运动信息。

section of a mixed nerve
Mixed nerve: long cord formed of nerve fibers, carrying sensory and motor messages between the central nervous system and the rest of the body.

皮肤
柔软且坚韧的器官。覆盖人体全身，具有保护、触觉感知和体温调节作用。

skin
Soft resistant organ covering the entire body, having roles of protection, tactile sensation and heat regulation.

神经外膜
包裹神经的结缔组织鞘。

epineurium
Sheath of connective tissue enveloping a nerve.

感受器
感觉器官中的细胞。当受到物理或化学刺激时能产生神经信息。

sensory receptor
Cell located in the sensory organs and capable of generating a nerve message when submitted to a physical or chemical stimulus.

神经束膜
包裹神经束的结缔组织鞘。

perineurium
Sheath of connective tissue enveloping a nerve fascicle.

神经纤维
运动神经或感觉神经的轴突。在神经内结成束状。

nerve fiber
Axon of a motor or sensory nerve, grouped into a fascicle inside a nerve.

感觉神经元
将感觉信息（如触觉、痛觉、温度）传递给中枢神经系统的神经元。

sensory neuron
Neuron transmitting sensory messages (such as touch, pain, temperature) to the central nervous system.

神经束
被神经束膜包裹的一组神经纤维。一条神经由若干神经束组成。

nerve fascicle
Group of nerve fibers surrounded by a sheath (perineurium); a nerve is formed of several nerve fascicles.

运动神经元
由中枢神经系统向肌肉和某些腺体传送神经冲动的神经元。

motor neuron
Neuron transmitting nerve impulses from the central nervous system to muscles and certain glands.

肌纤维
可收缩的细胞。肌肉的组成成分。

muscle fiber
Contractile cell, constituent element of muscles.

突触小体
轴突的最末端。与另一个细胞的膜形成突触。确保神经指令的传递。

synaptic knob
Extremity of an axon terminal forming a synapse with the membrane of another cell; it ensures transmission of nerve commands.

数百条神经 | Hundreds of Nerves

周围神经系统有31对脊神经和12对脑神经。这些神经又细分成无数的分支，支配着身体的各部位。
The peripheral nervous system has 31 pairs of spinal nerves and 12 pairs of cranial nerves, which subdivide into countless branches in order to innervate all parts of the body.

脑神经

从脑干发出的12对脑神经。为头部和颈部提供神经感知，并具有运动或感觉功能。

cranial nerves

Group of 12_pairs of nerves emerging from the brain stem, providing nerve sensation to the head and neck and serving a motor or sensory function.

脑下面观

脑：中枢神经系统的一部分。容纳于颅骨，包括大脑、小脑和脑干。

encephalon: inferior view

Encephalon: Part of the central nervous system contained in the skull, consisting of the cerebrum, cerebellum and brain stem.

嗅神经

感觉神经。负责嗅觉。

olfactory nerve
Sensory nerve involved in smell.

视神经

感觉神经：负责视觉，把信息从眼睛传送到脑。

optic nerve
Sensory nerve responsible for vision: it transmits information from the eye to the encephalon.

三叉神经

混合神经。将面部感觉传递到脑并参与咀嚼动作。

trigeminal nerve
Mixed nerve transmitting facial sensations to the encephalon and playing a role in chewing.

面神经

混合神经。控制面部运动和传送味觉。

facial nerve
Mixed nerve controlling facial movements and involved in taste sensations.

舌咽神经

混合神经。与吞咽，呕吐反射，味觉相关，并与舌头和咽部的部分感觉相关。

glossopharyngeal nerve
Mixed nerve associated with swallowing, gag reflex, taste and sensations from part of the tongue and pharynx.

动眼神经

运动神经。除了控制瞳孔的收缩，主要负责眼睛和上眼睑的运动。

oculomotor nerve
Motor nerve essentially responsible for eye and upper eyelid movements, as well as constriction of the pupil.

滑车神经

运动神经。主要参与眼球运动。

trochlear nerve
Motor nerve mainly involved in eye movements.

展神经

运动神经。控制眼球侧向运动。

abducent nerve
Motor nerve controlling lateral eye movements.

前庭蜗神经

感觉神经。负责听力和平衡。

vestibulocochlear nerve
Sensory nerve responsible for hearing and balance.

舌下神经

运动神经。主要控制舌头的运动，以便吞咽、咀嚼和说话。

hypoglossal nerve
Motor nerve mainly controlling the movement of the tongue to allow swallowing, chewing and talking.

副神经

运动神经。主要控制颈部运动和吞咽。

accessory nerve
Motor nerve essentially controlling neck movements and swallowing.

迷走神经

混合神经。支配所有脏器，在自主神经系统中起着重要作用。

vagus nerve
Mixed nerve playing an important role in the autonomic nervous system by innervating all the viscera.

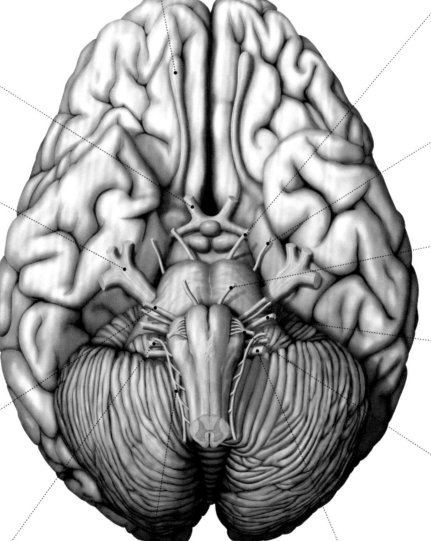

脊神经

31对起于脊髓的混合（感觉和运动）神经。支配人体除面部以外所有部分。

spinal nerves

Group of 31 pairs of mixed (sensory and motor) nerves emerging from the spinal cord, providing nerve sensations to all parts of the body, except the face.

笑容 | The Smile

微笑动作是面神经支配的，通过激活15块面部肌肉来完成。此神经的紊乱可能会导致人无法微笑（面瘫）。

The act of smiling is commanded by the facial nerve and activates some 15 muscles of the face. A disorder of this nerve may thus lead to an individual being unable to smile (facial paralysis).

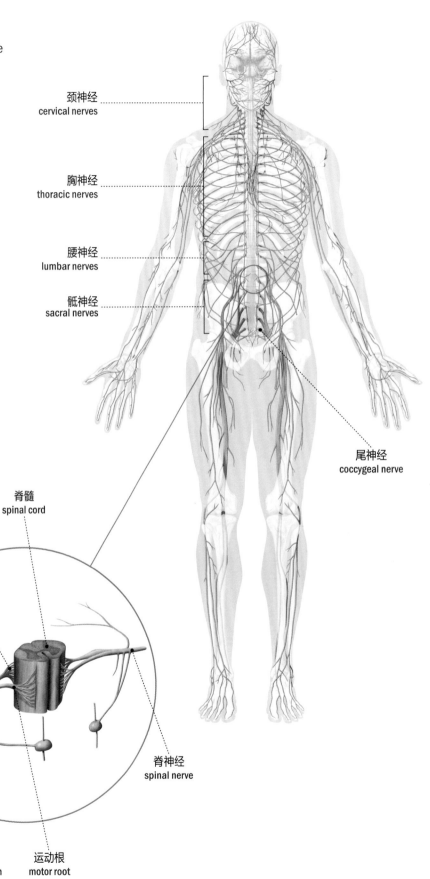

颈神经
cervical nerves

胸神经
thoracic nerves

腰神经
lumbar nerves

骶神经
sacral nerves

尾神经
coccygeal nerve

感觉根
sensory root

脊髓
spinal cord

脊神经节
spinal ganglion

后支
dorsal branch

前支
ventral branch

运动根
motor root

脊神经
spinal nerve

颈神经
支配头、颈、肩和上肢的8对脊神经。

cervical nerves
All eight pairs of spinal nerves innervating the head, neck, shoulders and upper limbs.

胸神经
支配胸部和背部的12对脊神经。

thoracic nerves
All 12 pairs of spinal nerves innervating the thorax and back.

腰神经
支配腹部和大腿的5对脊神经。

lumbar nerves
All five pairs of spinal nerves innervating the abdomen and thighs.

骶神经
支配下腹和下肢的5对脊神经。

sacral nerves
All five pairs of spinal nerves innervating the lower abdomen and lower limbs.

尾神经
支配尾骨区域的一对脊神经。

coccygeal nerve
Pair of spinal nerves innervating the coccyx region.

脊髓
中枢神经系统的一部分。位于脊柱内，负责将神经信息在脊神经和大脑之间来回传送。

spinal cord
Part of the central nervous system located in the vertebral column, transmitting nerve information from the spinal nerves to the brain and back.

脊神经
31对混合神经。包括感觉神经和运动神经，从脊髓发出。提供除面部以外身体所有部分的神经支配。

spinal nerve
Each of the mixed (sensory and motor) nerves emerging from the spinal cord and innervating all parts of the body, except the face.

感觉根
脊神经的一个分支。从身体的外周向脊髓传递感觉信息。

sensory root
Branch of a spinal nerve transmitting sensory information from the periphery of the body to the spinal cord.

运动根
脊神经的一个分支。将运动信息从脊髓传递到身体的外周，特别是肌肉组织。

motor root
Branch of a spinal nerve transmitting motor information from the spinal cord to the periphery of the body, especially the muscles.

脊神经节
由一组感觉神经元的细胞体组成的结节。

spinal ganglion
Nodule made up of a group of cell bodies of sensory neurons.

前支
脊神经的主要分支。支配四肢、躯干的前侧和外侧。

ventral branch
Main branch of the spinal nerve serving to innervate the limbs and anterior and lateral parts of the trunk.

后支
脊神经的主要分支，支配躯干后部的皮肤、肌肉、关节和骨骼。

dorsal branch
Main branch of a spinal nerve serving to innervate the skin, muscles, joints and bones of the posterior part of the trunk.

主要神经前面观

神经：由神经纤维组成的长索。在中枢神经系统和身体其他部分之间传递感觉信息或运动信息。

main nerves: anterior view

Nerve: long cord made up of nerve fibers, carrying sensory or motor messages between the central nervous system and the rest of the body.

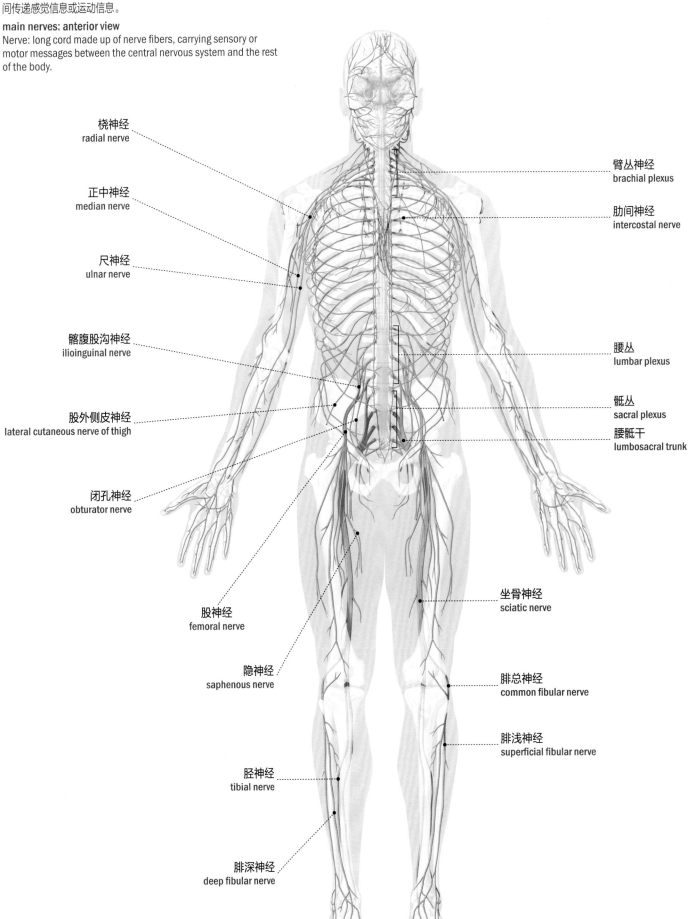

桡神经
radial nerve

正中神经
median nerve

尺神经
ulnar nerve

髂腹股沟神经
ilioinguinal nerve

股外侧皮神经
lateral cutaneous nerve of thigh

闭孔神经
obturator nerve

股神经
femoral nerve

隐神经
saphenous nerve

胫神经
tibial nerve

腓深神经
deep fibular nerve

臂丛神经
brachial plexus

肋间神经
intercostal nerve

腰丛
lumbar plexus

骶丛
sacral plexus

腰骶干
lumbosacral trunk

坐骨神经
sciatic nerve

腓总神经
common fibular nerve

腓浅神经
superficial fibular nerve

桡神经

起于臂丛的神经。主要支配上肢和手指的伸肌。

radial nerve
Nerve arising from the brachial plexus, innervating especially the extensor muscles of the upper limb and fingers.

正中神经

起源于臂丛的神经。支配前臂前部的肌肉，以及部分手部肌肉。

median nerve
Nerve arising from the brachial plexus, innervating various muscles of the anterior part of the forearm and part of the hand.

尺神经

起源于臂丛的神经。主要支配手和手指的屈肌。

ulnar nerve
Nerve arising from the brachial plexus, innervating especially the flexor muscles of the hand and fingers.

髂腹股沟神经

起于腰丛的神经。支配腹部、生殖器官和大腿等的部分区域。

ilioinguinal nerve
Nerve arising from the lumbar plexus, innervating part of the abdomen, genital organs and thigh.

股外侧皮神经

腰丛的分支。支配大腿外侧的皮肤。

lateral cutaneous nerve of thigh
Branch of the lumbar plexus innervating the skin of the outer part of the thigh.

闭孔神经

起于腰丛的神经。除了支配大腿的内侧区域，主要支配内收肌群。

obturator nerve
Nerve arising from the lumbar plexus, innervating mainly the adductor muscles, as well as the inner region of the thigh.

股神经

起于腰丛的神经。主要支配大腿屈肌和小腿伸肌。

femoral nerve
Nerve arising from the lumbar plexus, innervating especially the flexor muscles of the thigh and extensor muscles of the leg.

隐神经

股神经的分支。支配小腿和膝部的内侧。

saphenous nerve
Branch of the femoral nerve innervating the inner face of the leg and knee.

胫神经

坐骨神经的分支。支配部分小腿肌肉和足底。

tibial nerve
Branch of the sciatic nerve innervating certain leg muscles and the sole of the foot.

腓深神经

腓总神经的分支。主要支配小腿前部的肌肉和足背。

deep fibular nerve
Branch of the common fibular nerve innervating especially the muscles of the front part of the leg and back of the foot.

臂丛神经

神经丛。由后四根颈神经和第一根胸神经构成，其分支负责上肢的运动和感觉功能。

brachial plexus
Network of nerves formed by the last four cervical nerves and the first thoracic nerve; its branches ensure the motor skills and responsiveness of the upper limbs.

肋间神经

除了支配肋间肌，还支配部分膈肌和腹壁。

intercostal nerve
Each of the nerves innervating the intercostal muscles, as well as part of the diaphragm and abdominal wall.

腰丛

神经丛。由上四根腰神经构成，其分支负责下肢的运动和感觉功能。

lumbar plexus
Network of nerves formed by the first four lumbar nerves; its branches ensure the motor skills and responsiveness of the lower limbs.

骶丛

神经丛。由腰骶干和上3根骶神经构成，其分支支配臀部和部分大腿的运动和感觉功能。

sacral plexus
Network of nerves formed by the lumbosacral trunk and first three sacral nerves; its branches ensure the motor skills and responsiveness of the buttock and part of the thigh.

腰骶干

由第四和第五腰神经组成的神经。终于骶丛。

lumbosacral trunk
Nerve formed by the fourth and fifth lumbar nerves, ending at the sacral plexus.

坐骨神经

起于骶丛的神经。支配着下肢的大部分。

sciatic nerve
Nerve arising from the sacral plexus, innervating a large part of the lower limbs.

腓总神经

坐骨神经的分支。支配膝部和小腿前侧和外侧的肌肉。

common fibular nerve
Branch of the sciatic nerve innervating the knee and muscles of the anterior and lateral parts of the leg.

腓浅神经

腓总神经的分支。主要支配小腿的外侧和足背。

superficial fibular nerve
Branch of the common fibular nerve innervating especially the outer part of the leg and back of the foot.

神经系统 ｜ NERVOUS SYSTEM

前臂和手后面观
forearm and hand: posterior view

正中神经
median nerve

前臂骨间背神经
posterior interosseous nerve of forearm

桡神经
radial nerve

尺神经
ulnar nerve

指掌侧总神经
common palmar digital nerves

指掌侧固有神经
proper palmar digital nerves

腿后面观
leg: posterior view

股神经
femoral nerve

腓总神经
common fibular nerve

胫神经
tibial nerve

腓浅神经
superficial fibular nerve

腓深神经
deep fibular nerve

最长的神经 ｜ The Longest

坐骨神经是人体内最长、最粗的一条神经。它起于腰的下部，经由骨盆区向下延伸，沿着大腿，一直到小腿后侧。坐骨神经的某些部分直径能有大拇指那么粗。

The sciatic nerve is the longest and largest nerve in the body. Running from the bottom of the back through the pelvic region down the thigh and the back of the leg, it has a diameter as thick as a thumb in some places.

正中神经

起于臂丛的神经。支配前臂前侧的多个肌肉以及手的部分肌肉。

median nerve

Nerve arising from the brachial plexus, innervating various muscles of the anterior part of the forearm and part of the hand.

尺神经

起于臂丛的神经。主要支配手和手指的屈肌。

ulnar nerve

Nerve arising from the brachial plexus, innervating especially the flexor muscles of the hand and fingers.

前臂骨间背神经

桡神经的分支。主要支配前臂的伸肌。

posterior interosseous nerve of forearm

Branch of the radial nerve innervating mainly the extensor muscles of the forearm.

指掌侧总神经

正中神经的分支。支配手掌肌肉。

common palmar digital nerves

Branches of the median nerve innervating the muscles of the palm of the hand.

桡神经

起于臂丛的神经。主要支配上肢和手指的伸肌。

radial nerve

Nerve arising from the brachial plexus, innervating especially the extensor muscles of the upper limb and fingers.

指掌侧固有神经

掌侧指总神经的分支,支配手指。

proper palmar digital nerves

Branches of common palmar digital nerves innervating the fingers.

股神经

起于腰丛的神经,主要支配大腿屈肌和小腿伸肌。

femoral nerve

Nerve arising from the lumbar plexus, innervating especially the flexor muscles of the thigh and extensor muscles of the leg.

腓浅神经

腓总神经的分支。主要支配小腿外侧和足背。

superficial fibular nerve

Branch of the common fibular nerve innervating especially the outer part of the leg and back of the foot.

腓总神经

坐骨神经的分支。支配膝部和小腿前侧与外侧的肌肉。

common fibular nerve

Branch of the sciatic nerve innervating the knee and muscles of the anterior and lateral parts of the leg.

腓深神经

腓总神经的分支。主要支配小腿前部的肌肉和足背。

deep fibular nerve

Branch of the common fibular nerve innervating especially the muscles of the front part of the leg and back of the foot.

胫神经

坐骨神经的分支。支配部分小腿肌肉和足底。

tibial nerve

Branch of the sciatic nerve innervating certain leg muscles and the sole of the foot.

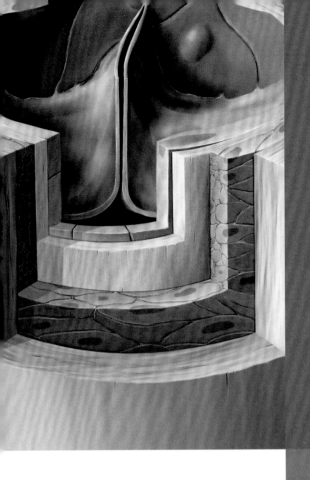

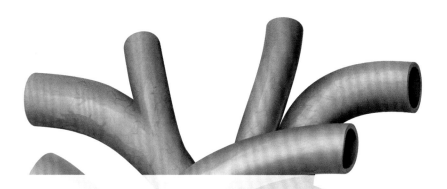

心血管系统 Cardiovascular system

心血管系统由多个器官组成，这些器官实现血液在体内的循环并使血液在肺部获氧。在心脏有规律收缩的推动下，血液进入动脉、毛细血管和静脉组成的网络。带去细胞所需的氧和各种营养物质，同时排走各种代谢产物，如二氧化碳。血液还能将激素和白细胞送达身体的大多数部位。

The cardiovascular system is the group of organs that circulate blood through the body and oxygenate blood in the lungs. Propelled by regular contractions of the heart, blood enters the network of arteries, capillaries, and veins to carry the oxygen and nutrients that cells need, and to drain various waste products, such as carbon dioxide. It also enables hormones and white blood cells to reach most parts of the body.

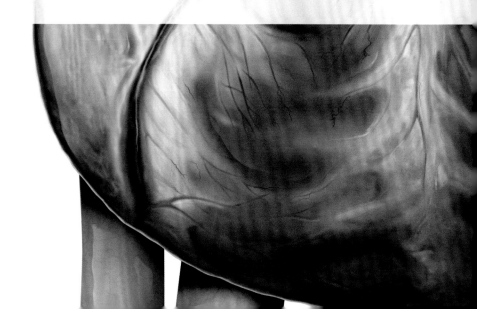

血液 | blood

血液

在血管中循环流动的红色黏性液体。血液循环由心脏推动。

blood
Viscous red fluid circulating in the blood vessels and propelled by the heart.

血液成分

血液是一种液体。由血浆及血细胞等成分组成，血细胞在血浆中流动。

composition of blood
Blood is made up of a liquid element (plasma) in which blood cells circulate.

白细胞
血细胞的一种。白细胞属于免疫系统，在机体防御疾病中发挥关键作用。

white blood cell
Blood cell belonging to the immune system and playing an essential role in the body's defenses.

血管
供血液循环流动的通道。血管分为动脉、毛细血管和静脉。

blood vessel
Channel through which blood circulates; there are arteries, capillaries and veins.

血浆
淡黄色液体。由水、营养物质、矿物质和蛋白质组成，血细胞在其中流动。血浆输送营养物质并将热量分布到全身。

plasma
Yellowish fluid made up of water, nutrients, minerals and proteins in which blood cells circulate; it transports nutrients and distributes warmth throughout the body.

血小板
血细胞的一种。能促进血液凝固从而防止出血。

platelet
Blood cell ensuring the coagulation of blood and preventing hemorrhages.

红细胞
血细胞的一种。能将氧气从肺输送到各个组织并将二氧化碳从各个组织输送回肺。

red blood cell
Blood cell that carries oxygen from the lungs to the tissues and carbon dioxide from the tissues to the lungs.

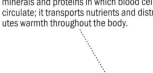

珠蛋白
血红蛋白中的蛋白质成分。

globin
Protein constituent of hemoglobin.

血细胞

血液中的细胞。包括红细胞、多种白细胞和血小板。

blood cells
Cells present in the blood, consisting of red blood cells, various types of white blood cells and platelets.

血红素
血红蛋白中的含铁分子。可以与氧分子结合。血红蛋白因血红素而呈红色。

heme
Molecule containing iron to which oxygen molecules bind; heme gives hemoglobin its red color.

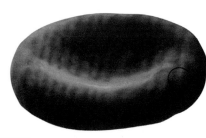

红细胞
血细胞的一种。能将氧气从肺输送到各个组织并将二氧化碳从各个组织输送回肺。

red blood cell
Blood cell that carries oxygen from the lungs to the tissues and carbon dioxide from the tissues to the lungs.

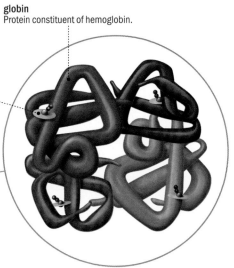

血红蛋白
红细胞内的复杂分子。能运送氧气和二氧化碳。

hemoglobin
Complex molecule contained in red blood cells, allowing oxygen and carbon dioxide to be transported.

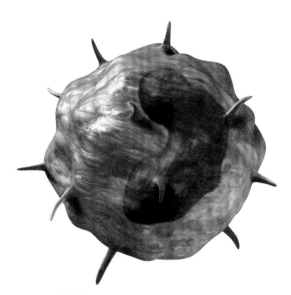

单核细胞
白细胞的一种，在组织的炎症过程中转化为巨噬细胞（可消灭细菌和吞噬死亡细胞的细胞）。

monocyte
White blood cell that transforms into a macrophage (cell that destroys bacteria and dead cells) in the tissues during inflammation.

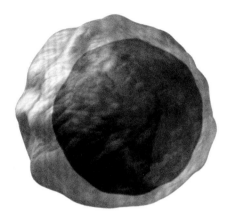

淋巴细胞
白细胞的一种。在免疫系统中起关键作用，尤其是能产生抗体。淋巴细胞在血管和淋巴器官中循环。

lymphocyte
White blood cell playing a fundamental role in the immune system, especially by producing antibodies; it circulates in blood vessels and lymphatic organs.

颗粒
球形小颗粒。含有各种化学物质，具有毒性或炎症特性。

granule
Small spherical particle containing various chemical substances having toxic or inflammatory properties.

颗粒
球形小颗粒。含有各种化学物质，参与血液凝固。

granule
Small spherical particle containing various chemical substances involved in the coagulation of blood.

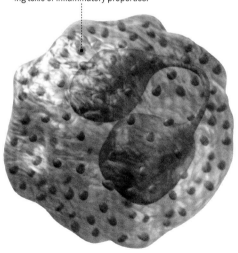

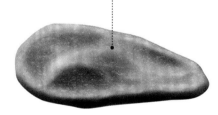

血小板
血细胞的一种。能促进血液凝固从而防止出血。

platelet
Blood cell ensuring the coagulation of blood and preventing hemorrhages.

粒细胞
白细胞的一种，单核分叶。参与炎症反应、消灭寄生虫和过敏反应。

granulocyte
White blood cell having a nucleus with several lobes; it is involved in the inflammatory reaction, destruction of parasites and allergic reactions.

人体血量不过几升而已 | A Few Liters of Blood

成人体内血液总量在4升至5升。一滴血中就含有2亿个红细胞。

The adult body contains a total of between 4 and 5 liters of blood. A single drop of blood contains 200 million red blood cells.

血液循环

血液在复杂血管网络内有规律和不间断的运动。血液循环分为两个不同的回路：肺循环和体循环。

blood circulation

Regular and constant movement of blood within the complex network of blood vessels divided into two distinct circuits: pulmonary circulation and systemic circulation.

肺循环

保障肺内血液和空气之间进行气体交换的所有血管。

pulmonary circulation

All the blood vessels ensuring gaseous exchanges between blood and air in the lungs.

动脉血

富含氧气的血液。在动脉、肺静脉和左心房、左心室循环。

arterial blood

Blood rich in oxygen circulating in the arteries, pulmonary veins and left cavities of the heart.

静脉血

含氧量低而含二氧化碳高的血液。在静脉、肺动脉和右心房、右心室循环。

venous blood

Blood poor in oxygen and rich in carbon dioxide, circulating in the veins, pulmonary arteries and right cavities of the heart.

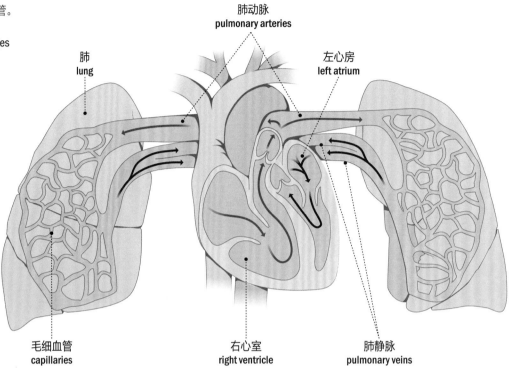

肺动脉
pulmonary arteries

肺
lung

左心房
left atrium

毛细血管
capillaries

右心室
right ventricle

肺静脉
pulmonary veins

体循环

保障身体各组织和各器官血液供应的所有血管。

systemic circulation

All the blood vessels ensuring blood irrigation of tissues and organs.

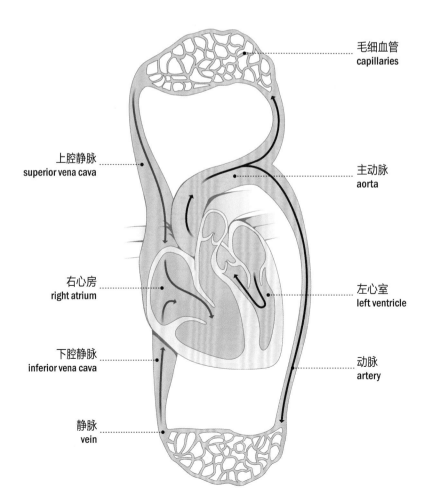

毛细血管
capillaries

上腔静脉
superior vena cava

主动脉
aorta

右心房
right atrium

左心室
left ventricle

下腔静脉
inferior vena cava

动脉
artery

静脉
vein

肺
呼吸器官。由弹性组织构成。负责空气和血液间的气体交换。

lung
Organ of the respiratory tract formed of extensible tissue and responsible for gaseous exchanges between air and blood.

毛细血管
确保小动脉和小静脉之间的血液循环的微小血管。肺毛细血管是血液与肺泡里的空气之间进行交换的场所。

capillaries
Tiny blood vessels ensuring blood circulation between an arteriole and a venule; the capillaries of the lungs are the site of gaseous exchanges between blood and air contained in the pulmonary alveoli.

肺动脉
把右心室排出的乏氧血输送到肺部的血管。

pulmonary arteries
Blood vessels carrying deoxygenated blood ejected by the right ventricle toward the lungs.

右心室
心腔之一。壁薄，接收来自右心房的乏氧血液，并将其推送到肺。

right ventricle
Thin-walled cavity of the heart receiving deoxygenated blood from the right atrium and propelling it to the lungs.

左心房
心腔之一。接收来自四个肺静脉的富氧血液，并将其推送进左心室。

left atrium
Cavity of the heart receiving oxygenated blood from the four pulmonary veins and propelling it into the left ventricle.

肺静脉
将富氧血从肺输送到左心房的静脉。

pulmonary veins
Veins carrying oxygenated blood from the lungs to the left atrium.

上腔静脉
将来自上半身（横膈膜上方）的乏氧血液输送至右心房的静脉。

superior vena cava
Vein carrying deoxygenated blood from the upper part of the body (above the diaphragm) to the right atrium of the heart.

毛细血管
确保小动脉和小静脉之间的血液循环的微小血管。肺毛细血管是血液与肺泡里的空气之间进行交换的场所。

capillaries
Tiny blood vessels ensuring blood circulation between an arteriole and a venule; they form the dense networks in which oxygen from the blood is transferred to the cells, and carbon dioxide from the cells is transferred to the blood.

右心房
心腔之一。从腔静脉接收乏氧血并将其推送进右心室。

right atrium
Cavity of the heart receiving deoxygenated blood from the venae cavae and propelling it into the right ventricle.

主动脉
人体的主要动脉。负责将左心室泵出的富氧血输送到全身器官。

aorta
Main artery of the body, carrying oxygenated blood ejected by the left ventricle to the organs.

下腔静脉
将来自下半身（横膈膜下方）的乏氧血液输送至右心房的静脉。

inferior vena cava
Vein carrying deoxygenated blood from the lower part of the body (below the diaphragm) to the right atrium of the heart.

左心室
心腔之一。壁厚，接收来自左心房的富氧血液，并将其推送进主动脉，以供应全身。

left ventricle
Thick-walled cavity of the heart receiving oxygenated blood from the left atrium and propelling it into the aorta to irrigate the body.

静脉
将血液从全身各器官输送回心脏的血管。

vein
Blood vessel carrying blood from the organs back to the heart.

动脉
将富氧血液由心脏输送到全身的血管。

artery
Blood vessel carrying oxygenated blood from the heart to all parts of the body.

血管 | blood vessels

血管
供血液循环流动的通道。血管分为动脉、毛细血管和静脉。

blood vessels
Canals through which blood circulates; there are arteries, capillaries and veins.

毛细血管截面
毛细血管：确保小动脉和小静脉之间血液循环的微小血管。它的管壁允许血液和毛细血管的外表面进行交换。

section of a capillary
Capillary: tiny blood vessel ensuring blood circulation between an arteriole and a venule; its wall allows exchanges between blood and the exterior surface of the capillary.

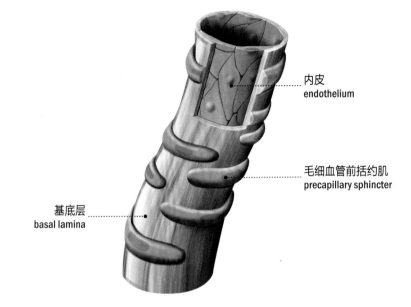

内皮
endothelium

毛细血管前括约肌
precapillary sphincter

基底层
basal lamina

动脉截面
动脉：将富氧血液从心脏输送到全身的血管。动脉管壁富含平滑肌和弹性纤维，其口径因此可变，能调控血液的流通。

section of an artery
Artery: blood vessel carrying oxygenated blood from the heart to all parts of the body; its wall, rich in smooth muscles and elastic fibers, adjusts in size to regulate circulation.

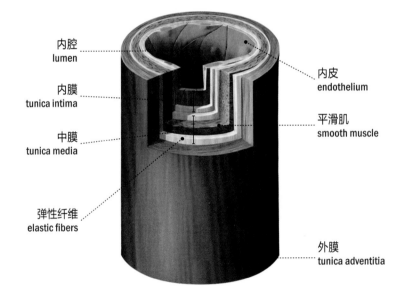

内腔
lumen

内膜
tunica intima

中膜
tunica media

弹性纤维
elastic fibers

内皮
endothelium

平滑肌
smooth muscle

外膜
tunica adventitia

静脉截面
静脉：将乏氧血从各个器官输送回心脏的血管。静脉的管壁比动脉的要薄。

section of a vein
Vein: blood vessel carrying deoxygenated blood from the organs back to the heart; veins have thinner walls than arteries.

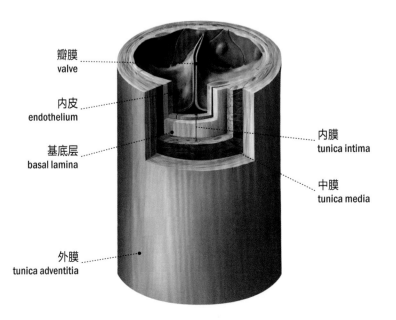

瓣膜
valve

内皮
endothelium

基底层
basal lamina

内膜
tunica intima

中膜
tunica media

外膜
tunica adventitia

直径不一 | Variable Diameter

血管能够通过缩小口径（血管收缩）或扩大口径（血管舒张）来调节血液流动。这种现象在中等直径的动脉和小动脉中特别明显。

The blood vessels are able to reduce their caliber (vasoconstriction) or increase it (vasodilation) in order to regulate blood flow. This phenomenon is particularly apparent in arteries of medium diameter and the arterioles.

基底层
附着在内皮上的薄薄的膜。
basal lamina
Fine membrane adhering to the endothelium.

内皮
上皮组织。被覆于毛细血管的内表面。
endothelium
Epithelial tissue lining the interior surface of the capillary.

毛细血管前括约肌
环状肌肉纤维。包裹毛细血管壁周围，可不自主地收缩和舒张，以调节血液流动。
precapillary sphincter
Ring-shaped muscle fiber surrounding the wall of a blood capillary, involuntarily contracting and releasing to regulate blood flow.

内腔
空腔器官的中间开口。
lumen
Central opening of a hollow organ.

内膜
血管的内层。由内皮和基底膜构成。
tunica intima
Inner layer of a blood vessel made of an endothelium and a basal lamina.

中膜
动静脉管壁的中间层。由平滑肌和弹性纤维构成。
tunica media
Middle layer of the wall of the arteries and veins, made of smooth muscles and elastic fibers.

弹性纤维
主要由弹性蛋白构成的纤维。弹性蛋白是一种能够拉伸然后恢复其原始形状的蛋白质。
elastic fibers
Fibers mostly made of elastin, a protein capable of stretching and then returning to its original shape.

内皮
上皮组织。被覆于动脉的内表面。
endothelium
Epithelial tissue lining the interior surface of the artery.

平滑肌
肌肉的一种。在自主神经系统或激素作用下，可使某些器官做不自主的运动。
smooth muscle
Muscle allowing involuntary movements of certain organs, in response to action of the autonomic nervous system or hormones.

外膜
动静脉管壁的外层。富含胶原纤维。
tunica adventitia
Outer layer of the wall of the arteries and veins, rich in collagen fibers.

瓣膜
静脉内的膜状折叠。以防止血液倒流。
valve
Membranous fold inside a vein, preventing reverse blood flow.

内皮
上皮组织。被覆于静脉的内表面。
endothelium
Epithelial tissue lining the interior surface of the vein.

基底层
确保上皮细胞能黏附于比邻组织的膜。
basal lamina
Membrane ensuring the adherence of epithelial cells to adjacent tissue.

外膜
动静脉管壁的外层。富含胶原纤维。
tunica adventitia
Outer layer of the wall of the arteries and veins, rich in collagen fibers.

内膜
血管的内层。由内皮和基底膜构成。
tunica intima
Inner layer of a blood vessel made of an endothelium and a basal lamina.

中膜
动静脉管壁的中间层。由平滑肌和弹性纤维构成。
tunica media
Middle layer of the wall of the arteries and veins, made of smooth muscles and elastic fibers.

主要动脉前面观

动脉：将富氧血液从心脏输送到全身的血管。大多数动脉都是成对出现的，分别供应身体的左侧和右侧。

principal arteries: anterior view

Artery: blood vessel carrying oxygenated blood from the heart to all parts of the body; most arteries present as two copies that irrigate the left and right sides of the body.

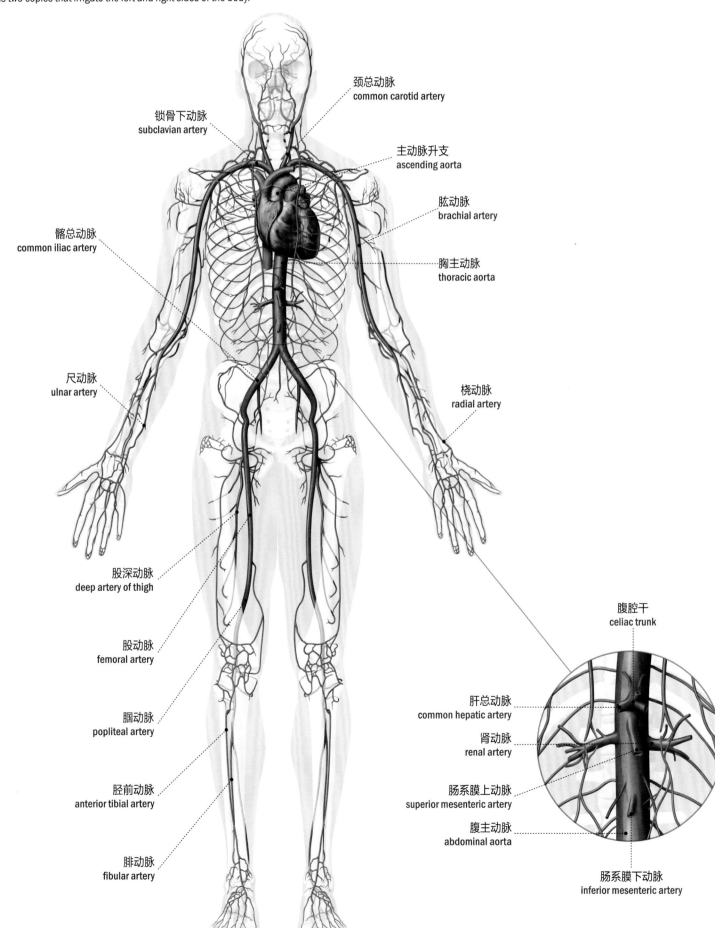

颈总动脉
common carotid artery

锁骨下动脉
subclavian artery

主动脉升支
ascending aorta

肱动脉
brachial artery

胸主动脉
thoracic aorta

髂总动脉
common iliac artery

尺动脉
ulnar artery

桡动脉
radial artery

股深动脉
deep artery of thigh

股动脉
femoral artery

腘动脉
popliteal artery

胫前动脉
anterior tibial artery

腓动脉
fibular artery

腹腔干
celiac trunk

肝总动脉
common hepatic artery

肾动脉
renal artery

肠系膜上动脉
superior mesenteric artery

腹主动脉
abdominal aorta

肠系膜下动脉
inferior mesenteric artery

颈总动脉

供应头部和上颈部的动脉。分为颈外动脉和颈内动脉。

common carotid artery

Artery irrigating the head and upper part of the neck; it is divided into outer and inner carotid arteries.

锁骨下动脉

上肢的主要动脉。穿过锁骨下方，也供应下颈部。

subclavian artery

Main artery of the upper limbs, passing beneath the clavicle; it also irrigates the lower part of the neck.

髂总动脉

腹主动脉的两个末端分支。每个末端分支都分为髂外动脉和髂内动脉。

common iliac artery

Each of two terminal branches of the abdominal artery that divide into the external and internal iliac arteries.

尺动脉

肱动脉末端分支。主要供应前臂的后部。

ulnar artery

Terminal branch of the brachial artery, irrigating mainly the posterior part of the forearm.

股深动脉

股动脉的分支。供应大腿的肌肉、髋部和股骨。

deep artery of thigh

Branch of the femoral artery irrigating the muscles of the thigh, hip region and femur.

股动脉

大腿的主要动脉。沿股骨内侧向下延伸。

femoral artery

Main artery of the thigh, running along the inner side of the femur.

腘动脉

股动脉的延伸。供应膝关节和小腿区域。

popliteal artery

Extension of the femoral artery, irrigating the regions of the knee and calf.

胫前动脉

腘动脉的分支。沿着小腿的前侧延伸并供应伸肌。

anterior tibial artery

Branch of the popliteal artery running along the anterior side of the leg and irrigating the extensor muscles.

腓动脉

胫骨后动脉分支。供应小腿的肌肉和踝关节区域。

fibular artery

Branch of the posterior tibial artery irrigating the muscles of the calf and ankle region.

主动脉升支

主动脉的第一段。从左心室开始分出两条冠状动脉，供应心脏。

ascending aorta

First segment of the aorta, starting from the left ventricle and giving rise to two coronary arteries irrigating the heart.

肱动脉

沿肱骨延伸的动脉。供应上臂的屈肌，终止于肘部，并分为两支（桡动脉和尺动脉）。

brachial artery

Artery running along the humerus and irrigating the flexor muscles of the arm; it ends at the elbow, dividing into two branches (the radial artery and the ulnar artery).

胸主动脉

主动脉的第三段。在胸腔降至隔膜，并形成位于肋骨之间的多个动脉分支（肋间动脉，肋下动脉）。

thoracic aorta

Third segment of the aorta, descending in the thorax to the diaphragm and giving rise to various arteries located between the ribs (intercostal arteries, subcostal artery).

桡动脉

肱动脉的终末分支。供应前臂和腕前部的肌肉。

radial artery

Terminal branch of the brachial artery, irrigating the muscles of the anterior part of the forearm and carpus.

腹腔干

腹主动脉的分支。分为三根动脉，以供应腹部器官。

celiac trunk

Branch of the abdominal aorta dividing into three arteries to serve the organs of the abdomen.

肝总动脉

腹腔干的分支。主要用于供应肝脏。

common hepatic artery

Branch of the celiac trunk serving mainly to irrigate the liver.

肾动脉

腹主动脉分支。供应肾脏。

renal artery

Branch of the abdominal aorta irrigating the kidney.

肠系膜上动脉

腹主动脉的分支。供应部分肠道（小肠，右结肠）。

superior mesenteric artery

Branch of the abdominal aorta irrigating part of the intestines (small intestine, right colon).

腹主动脉

主动脉的第四段。也是最后一段。向下进入腹腔并形成多个分支，主要通向肾脏、胰腺和结肠。

abdominal aorta

Fourth and last segment of the aorta, passing down into the abdominal cavity and giving rise to various arteries leading especially toward the kidneys, pancreas and colon.

肠系膜下动脉

腹主动脉的分支。供应低位结肠和横结肠的一半。

inferior mesenteric artery

Branch of the abdominal aorta irrigating the large lower intestine and half the transverse colon.

主要静脉前面观
principal veins: anterior view

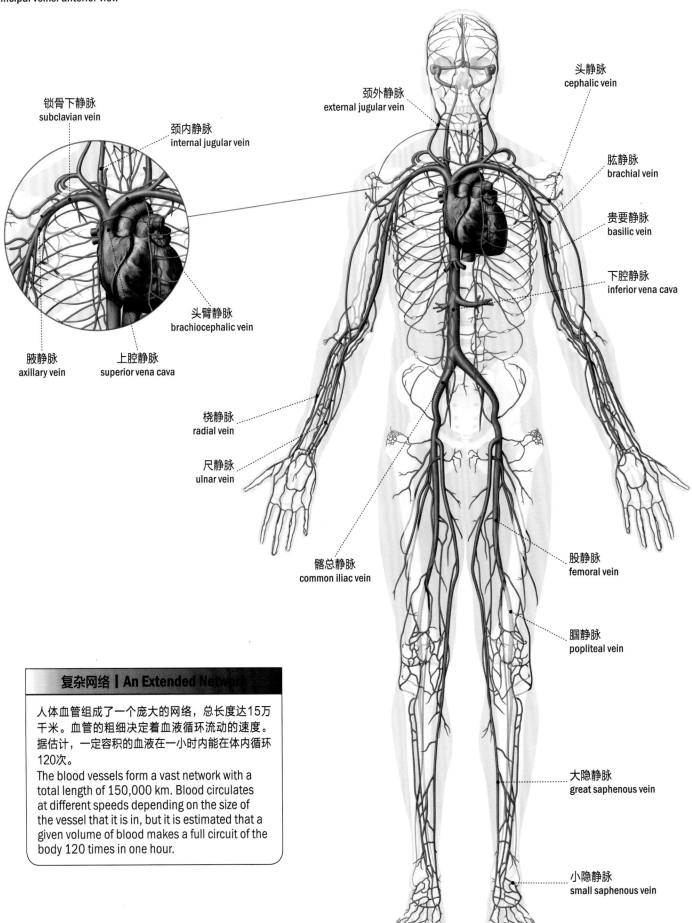

锁骨下静脉
subclavian vein

颈内静脉
internal jugular vein

颈外静脉
external jugular vein

头静脉
cephalic vein

肱静脉
brachial vein

贵要静脉
basilic vein

下腔静脉
inferior vena cava

头臂静脉
brachiocephalic vein

腋静脉
axillary vein

上腔静脉
superior vena cava

桡静脉
radial vein

尺静脉
ulnar vein

髂总静脉
common iliac vein

股静脉
femoral vein

腘静脉
popliteal vein

大隐静脉
great saphenous vein

小隐静脉
small saphenous vein

复杂网络 | An Extended Network

人体血管组成了一个庞大的网络，总长度达15万千米。血管的粗细决定着血液循环流动的速度。据估计，一定容积的血液在一小时内能在体内循环120次。

The blood vessels form a vast network with a total length of 150,000 km. Blood circulates at different speeds depending on the size of the vessel that it is in, but it is estimated that a given volume of blood makes a full circuit of the body 120 times in one hour.

主要静脉前面观

静脉：将乏氧血从各个器官输送回心脏的血管。大多数静脉成对出现，分别回输身体左右两侧的乏氧血。

principal veins: anterior view

Vein: blood vessel carrying deoxygenated blood from the organs back to the heart; most veins present as two copies that drain the left and right parts of the body.

锁骨下静脉

腋静脉的延伸。收集手臂，部分颈部和面部的血液，它与颈内静脉汇合形成头臂静脉。

subclavian vein

Extension of the axillary vein collecting the blood of the arm and part of the neck and face; it joins the internal jugular vein to form the brachiocephalic vein.

颈内静脉

收集脑部、部分面部和颈部血液的静脉。和锁骨下静脉汇合形成头臂静脉。

internal jugular vein

Vein draining the blood of the encephalon, part of the face and neck; it joins the subclavian vein to form the brachiocephalic vein.

头臂静脉

收集头部、颈部和上肢血液的静脉。有两条。

brachiocephalic vein

Each of two veins collecting the blood of the head, neck and upper limbs.

上腔静脉

将来自身体上部（横膈膜上方）的乏氧血输送至右心房的静脉。

superior vena cava

Vein carrying deoxygenated blood from the upper part of the body (above the diaphragm) to the right atrium of the heart.

腋静脉

静脉。穿过腋窝凹陷处，最终止于锁骨下静脉，主要接受来自肩部和胸部的静脉。

axillary vein

Vein crossing the hollow of the armpit and ending at the subclavian vein; it receives especially the veins of the shoulder and thorax.

颈外静脉

起于腮腺区域的静脉。最终汇入锁骨下静脉。

external jugular vein

Vein originating in the region of the parotid gland and entering the subclavian vein.

桡静脉

接收手部血液回流的静脉。参与构成肱静脉。

radial vein

Vein receiving the blood of the hand and then assisting in forming the brachial vein.

尺静脉

前臂后部的静脉。在肘部与桡静脉汇合形成肱静脉。

ulnar vein

Vein of the posterior part of the forearm, joining with the radial vein at the elbow to form the brachial vein.

髂总静脉

将下肢和骨盆的血液输送到下腔静脉的静脉。

common iliac vein

Vein carrying the blood of the lower limbs and pelvis to the inferior vena cava.

头静脉

上臂外侧静脉。下降汇入腋静脉，汇集肩部的浅静脉。

cephalic vein

Vein of the outer side of the arm, descending into the axillary vein; it receives the superficial veins of the shoulder.

肱静脉

上臂的静脉。与贵要静脉汇合形成腋静脉。

brachial vein

Vein of the arm joining with the basilic vein to form the axillary vein.

贵要静脉

上臂内侧的静脉。与肱静脉汇合形成腋静脉。

basilic vein

Vein of the inner side of the arm joining with the brachial veins to form the axillary vein.

下腔静脉

将来自身体下部（横膈膜下方）的乏氧血输送至右心房的静脉。

inferior vena cava

Vein carrying deoxygenated blood from the lower part of the body (below the diaphragm) to the right atrium of the heart.

股静脉

腘静脉的延伸。收集大腿深部区域的乏氧血。进入腹部后，成为髂外静脉。

femoral vein

Extension of the popliteal vein, draining the deep regions of the thigh; as it enters the abdomen, it becomes the external iliac vein.

腘静脉

由胫前和胫后静脉汇合形成的静脉。延伸至股静脉。

popliteal vein

Vein formed by the union of the posterior and anterior tibial veins and extending via the femoral vein.

大隐静脉

汇集小腿和大腿内侧的血液的静脉。并接收部分足部静脉血。是人体最长的静脉。

great saphenous vein

Vein collecting the blood of the medial side of the leg and thigh and receiving certain veins of the foot. It is the longest vein in the body.

小隐静脉

起自足外侧的静脉。在膝部重新汇入腘静脉。

small saphenous vein

Vein originating in the lateral part of the foot and rejoining the popliteal vein at the knee.

头颈部前面观
head and neck: anterior view

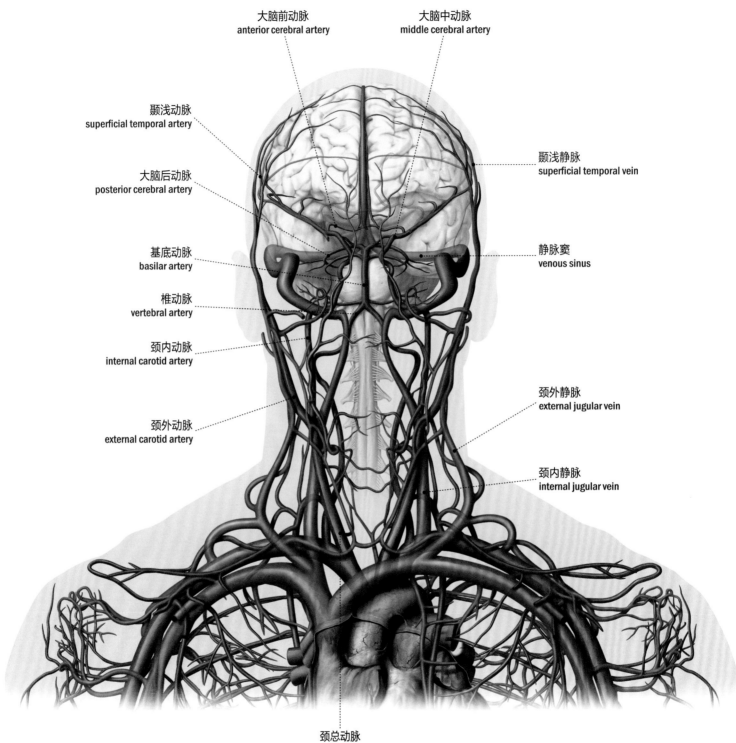

大脑前动脉
anterior cerebral artery

大脑中动脉
middle cerebral artery

颞浅动脉
superficial temporal artery

大脑后动脉
posterior cerebral artery

基底动脉
basilar artery

椎动脉
vertebral artery

颈内动脉
internal carotid artery

颈外动脉
external carotid artery

颞浅静脉
superficial temporal vein

静脉窦
venous sinus

颈外静脉
external jugular vein

颈内静脉
internal jugular vein

颈总动脉
common carotid artery

新鲜血液 | New Blood

心脏泵出的血液中约有20%，或者说每分钟就有近1升的血液流向脑。其中有部分血液被过滤后产生脑脊液。脑就包围在脑脊液中。

About 20% of the blood pumped by the heart, or almost one liter of blood per minute, goes to the brain. Part of this blood is filtered to produce cephaloradichian liquid, in which the brain floats.

心血管系统 | CARDIOVASCULAR SYSTEM

大脑前动脉
颈内动脉的分支。供应额叶和部分胼胝体。

anterior cerebral artery
Branch of the internal carotid artery irrigating the frontal lobe and part of the corpus callosum.

大脑中动脉
颈内动脉的分支。供应额叶、颞叶和顶叶的一部分。

middle cerebral artery
Branch of the internal carotid artery irrigating part of the frontal, temporal and parietal lobes.

颞浅动脉
颈外动脉的分支。主要供应额颞部。

superficial temporal artery
Branch of the external carotid artery irrigating mainly the temple region.

颞浅静脉
回流额颞部血液的静脉。

superficial temporal vein
Vein draining the blood of the temple region.

大脑后动脉
基底动脉的末端分支。供应颞叶和枕叶的下部。

posterior cerebral artery
Terminal branch of the basilar artery, irrigating the lower side of the temporal and occipital lobes.

静脉窦
在两层硬脑膜之间循环的静脉。将脑的血液回流到颈内静脉。

venous sinus
Vein circulating between two layers of dura mater and draining the blood of the encephalon toward the internal jugular vein.

基底动脉
由两个椎动脉汇合而成，然后分支形成大脑后动脉。

basilar artery
Artery resulting from the union of two vertebral arteries and then dividing to form the posterior cerebral arteries.

颈外静脉
起于腮腺区域的静脉。最终汇入锁骨下静脉。

external jugular vein
Vein originating in the region of the parotid gland and entering the subclavian vein.

椎动脉
锁骨下动脉的分支。供应颈部肌肉、脑膜、脑干和小脑。

vertebral artery
Branch of the subclavian artery irrigating the neck muscles, meninges, brain stem and cerebellum.

颈内动脉
颈总动脉的分支。生成供应小脑和眼球的各级动脉。

internal carotid artery
Branch of the common carotid artery giving rise to various arteries irrigating the cerebellum and ocular globe.

颈内静脉
回流脑部、部分面部和颈部血液的静脉。与锁骨下静脉汇合，形成头臂静脉。

internal jugular vein
Vein draining the blood of the encephalon, part of the face and neck; it joins the subclavian vein to form the brachiocephalic vein.

颈外动脉
颈总动脉的分支。生成供应颈部和面部的各级动脉。

external carotid artery
Branch of the common carotid artery giving rise to various arteries irrigating the neck and face.

颈总动脉
供应头部和上颈部的动脉。分支为颈外动脉和颈内动脉。

common carotid artery
Artery irrigating the head and upper part of the neck; it is divided into outer and inner carotid arteries.

前臂和手前面观
forearm and hand: anterior view

尺静脉
ulnar vein

尺动脉
ulnar artery

桡动脉
radial artery

桡静脉
radial vein

掌深弓
deep palmar arch

掌浅弓
superficial palmar arch

掌浅静脉弓
superficial palmar venous arch

指掌侧静脉
palmar digital veins

指掌侧固有动脉
proper palmar digital arteries

足和腿前面观
foot and leg: anterior view

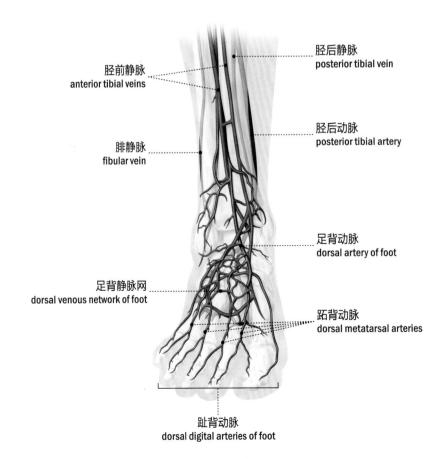

胫后静脉
posterior tibial vein

胫前静脉
anterior tibial veins

胫后动脉
posterior tibial artery

腓静脉
fibular vein

足背动脉
dorsal artery of foot

足背静脉网
dorsal venous network of foot

跖背动脉
dorsal metatarsal arteries

趾背动脉
dorsal digital arteries of foot

桡动脉
肱动脉的终末分支。供应前臂和腕前部的肌肉。

radial artery
Terminal branch of the brachial artery, irrigating the muscles of the anterior part of the forearm and carpus.

尺静脉
前臂后部的静脉。在肘部与桡静脉汇合形成肱静脉。

ulnar vein
Vein of the posterior part of the forearm, joining with the radial vein at the elbow to form the brachial vein.

桡静脉
接收手部回流血液的静脉。然后参与构成肱静脉。

radial vein
Vein receiving the blood of the hand and then assisting in forming the brachial vein.

尺动脉
肱动脉末端分支。主要供应前臂的后部。

ulnar artery
Terminal branch of the brachial artery, irrigating mainly the posterior part of the forearm.

掌深弓
手掌的动脉。由尺动脉的一个分支和桡动脉的末端汇合而成。

deep palmar arch
Artery of the palm of the hand formed by the union of a branch of the ulnar artery and the terminal end of the radial artery.

掌浅弓
手掌的动脉。由尺动脉和桡动脉的一个分支汇合而成。

superficial palmar arch
Artery of the palm of the hand, formed by the union of the ulnar artery and a branch of the radial artery.

掌浅静脉弓
静脉。接收手掌和手指血液回流，回流的血液随后进入尺静脉和桡静脉。

superficial palmar venous arch
Vessel receiving the veins of the palm of the hand and fingers; the blood it collects then passes into the ulnar and radial veins.

指掌侧静脉
手指的静脉。止于掌浅静脉弓。

palmar digital veins
Veins of the fingers ending at the superficial palmar venous arch.

指掌侧固有动脉
供应手指末端的小动脉。

proper palmar digital arteries
Small arteries irrigating the end of the fingers.

胫前静脉
小腿前侧的静脉。与胫后静脉汇合形成腘静脉。

anterior tibial veins
Veins of the anterior side of the leg, joining with the posterior tibial veins to form the popliteal vein.

胫后静脉
小腿后侧的静脉。与胫前静脉汇合形成腘静脉。

posterior tibial vein
Vein of the posterior side of the leg, joining with the anterior tibial veins to form the popliteal vein.

腓静脉
沿脚踝和部分小腿一直延伸到胫后静脉的静脉。

fibular vein
Vein running along the ankle and part of the leg to the posterior tibial veins.

胫后动脉
腘动脉的终末支。沿小腿后间隙下行，供应小腿和足底。

posterior tibial artery
Terminal branch of the popliteal artery running down the posterior compartment of the leg and irrigating the leg and sole of the foot.

足背静脉网
足背的浅静脉。汇入大隐静脉和小隐静脉。

dorsal venous network of foot
Superficial veins of the dorsum of the foot, entering the large and small saphenous veins.

足背动脉
胫前动脉的延伸。供应踝部和足背。

dorsal artery of foot
Extension of the anterior tibial artery irrigating the ankle and dorsum of the foot.

趾背动脉
供应足趾背侧的小动脉。

dorsal digital arteries of foot
Small arteries irrigating the dorsum of the toes.

跖背动脉
供应足趾的动脉。

dorsal metatarsal arteries
Arteries irrigating the toes.

心脏 | heart

心脏

肌性器官。分成四个腔，其可自主且有节奏地收缩，推动着血液在全身循环。

heart

Muscular organ divided into four chambers whose autonomous rhythmic contractions cause blood to circulate throughout the body.

心脏前剖面
frontal section of heart

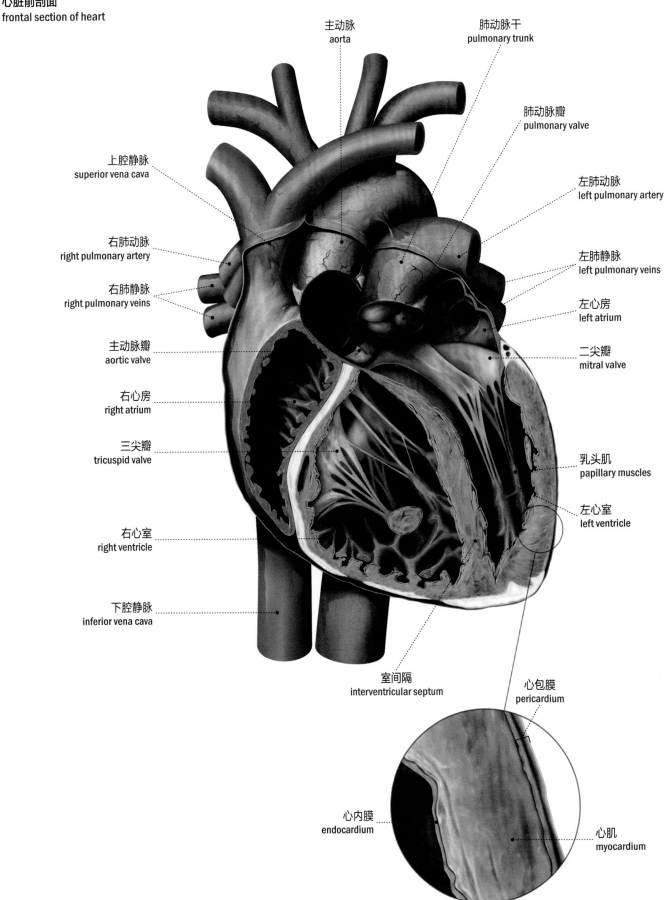

主动脉
aorta

肺动脉干
pulmonary trunk

肺动脉瓣
pulmonary valve

上腔静脉
superior vena cava

左肺动脉
left pulmonary artery

右肺动脉
right pulmonary artery

左肺静脉
left pulmonary veins

右肺静脉
right pulmonary veins

左心房
left atrium

主动脉瓣
aortic valve

二尖瓣
mitral valve

右心房
right atrium

三尖瓣
tricuspid valve

乳头肌
papillary muscles

左心室
left ventricle

右心室
right ventricle

下腔静脉
inferior vena cava

室间隔
interventricular septum

心包膜
pericardium

心内膜
endocardium

心肌
myocardium

主动脉
人体的主要动脉。负责将左心室泵出的富氧血输送到全身各器官。

aorta
Main artery of the body, carrying oxygenated blood ejected by the left ventricle to the organs.

上腔静脉
将来自身体上部（横膈膜上方）的乏氧血液输送至右心房的静脉。

superior vena cava
Vein carrying deoxygenated blood from the upper part of the body (above the diaphragm) to the right atrium of the heart.

右肺动脉
肺动脉干的分支。向右肺运送乏氧血液。

right pulmonary artery
Branch of the pulmonary trunk carrying deoxygenated blood to the right lung.

右肺静脉
将右肺中的富氧血液输送回左心房的静脉。

right pulmonary veins
Veins returning the oxygenated blood in the right lung to the left atrium of the heart.

主动脉瓣
弹性瓣膜结构。将血液从左心室输送到主动脉，并防止血液回流。

aortic valve
Elastic structure carrying the blood from the left ventricle to the aorta and preventing it from flowing back.

右心房
心腔之一。从腔静脉接受乏氧血，并推送入右心室。

right atrium
Cavity of the heart receiving deoxygenated blood from the venae cavae and propelling it into the right ventricle.

三尖瓣
弹性瓣膜结构。防止右心室的血液回流至右心房。

tricuspid valve
Elastic structure preventing the blood of the right ventricle from flowing back to the right atrium.

右心室
薄壁的心腔。接收来自右心房的乏氧血，并推送到肺动脉干。

right ventricle
Thin-walled chamber of the heart, receiving deoxygenated blood from the right atrium and propelling it into the pulmonary trunk toward the lungs.

下腔静脉
将来自身体下部（横膈膜下方）的乏氧血液输送到右心房的静脉。

inferior vena cava
Vein carrying deoxygenated blood from the lower part of the body (below the diaphragm) to the right atrium of the_heart.

心内膜
被覆于心脏各房室腔内表面的内皮，并与出入心脏的血管内皮相延续。

endocardium
Endothelium lining the interior surface of the chambers of the heart; it extends via the endothelium of the blood vessels connected to the heart.

肺动脉干
从右心室向两肺动脉输送血液的血管。

pulmonary trunk
Blood vessel carrying blood from the right ventricle to the two pulmonary arteries.

肺动脉瓣
弹性瓣膜结构。将血液从右心室输送到肺干，并防止血液回流。

pulmonary valve
Elastic structure carrying blood from the right ventricle to the pulmonary trunk and preventing its backflow.

左肺动脉
肺动脉干的分支。向左肺运送乏氧血液。

left pulmonary artery
Branch of the pulmonary trunk carrying deoxygenated blood to the left lung.

左肺静脉
将左肺中的富氧血液输送回左心房的静脉。

left pulmonary veins
Veins returning the oxygenated blood in the left lung to the left atrium of the heart.

左心房
心腔之一。从四条肺静脉接收富氧血，并推送入左心室。

left atrium
Cavity of the heart receiving oxygenated blood from the four pulmonary veins and propelling it into the left ventricle.

二尖瓣
弹性瓣膜结构。防止左心室的血液回流至左心房。

mitral valve
Elastic structure preventing the blood of the left ventricle from flowing back to the left atrium.

乳头肌
限制二尖瓣或三尖瓣的运动的肌肉，并防止瓣膜在心室收缩期间被推回到心房。

papillary muscles
Muscles limiting movement of the mitral or tricuspid valve and preventing it from being pushed back into the atrium during contraction of the ventricle.

左心室
厚壁的心腔。接收来自左心房的富氧血，并推送进主动脉，以供全身。

left ventricle
Thick-walled cavity of the heart receiving oxygenated blood from the left atrium and propelling it into the aorta to irrigate the body.

室间隔
主要由肌肉组成的壁。作用是将心脏的左右心室隔开。

interventricular septum
Mainly muscular wall separating the right and left ventricles of the heart.

心包膜
由多层结缔组织组成的包膜，包裹并保护心脏。

pericardium
Envelope of connective tissue formed of several layers, surrounding and protecting the heart.

心肌
厚实的肌肉层，包裹着心脏。可控制心脏收缩。

myocardium
Thick, muscular envelope of the heart, controlling cardiac contractions.

心脏前面观
heart: anterior view

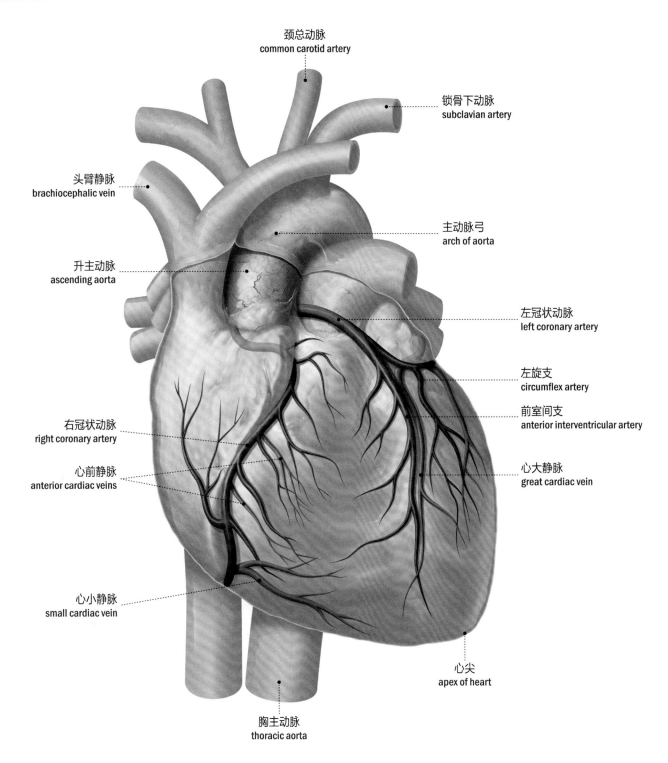

颈总动脉
common carotid artery

锁骨下动脉
subclavian artery

头臂静脉
brachiocephalic vein

主动脉弓
arch of aorta

升主动脉
ascending aorta

左冠状动脉
left coronary artery

左旋支
circumflex artery

前室间支
anterior interventricular artery

右冠状动脉
right coronary artery

心前静脉
anterior cardiac veins

心大静脉
great cardiac vein

心小静脉
small cardiac vein

心尖
apex of heart

胸主动脉
thoracic aorta

心动周期 | The Cardiac Cycle

心动周期是指心脏将血液推送进各级动脉的一系列活动过程。成人的心动周期平均持续0.8秒，泵出70毫升血液。心脏平均每分钟收缩70次，每天泵出约7 000升血液。
The cardiac cycle is the sequence of events enabling the heart to propel blood into the arteries. A cardiac cycle lasts an average of 0.8 seconds in adults and expels 70 ml of blood. The heart contracts an average of 70 times a minute, pumping some 7,000 liters of blood every day.

颈总动脉
供应头部和上颈的动脉。分为颈外动脉和颈内动脉。

common carotid artery
Artery irrigating the head and upper part of the neck; it is divided into outer and inner carotid arteries.

锁骨下动脉
上肢主要的动脉。穿过锁骨下方，也供应下颈部。

subclavian artery
Main artery of the upper limbs, passing beneath the clavicle; it also irrigates the lower part of the neck.

头臂静脉
汇集来自头部、颈部和上肢的血液的两条静脉。汇合形成上腔静脉。

brachiocephalic vein
Each of two veins collecting the blood of the head, neck and upper limbs and joining to form the superior vena cava.

主动脉弓
主动脉的第二段。形成多条动脉，供应头部和上肢。

arch of aorta
Second segment of the aorta, giving rise to the arteries irrigating the head and upper limbs.

升主动脉
主动脉的第一段。起于左心室，发出两条冠状动脉供应心脏。

ascending aorta
First segment of the aorta, starting from the left ventricle and giving rise to two coronary arteries irrigating the heart.

左冠状动脉
起于主动脉的动脉。供应心脏的左侧。

left coronary artery
Artery originating in the aorta and irrigating the left side of the heart.

右冠状动脉
起于主动脉的动脉。供应心脏的右侧。

right coronary artery
Artery originating in the aorta and irrigating the right side of the heart.

左旋支
左冠状动脉的末端分支。供应左心室和左心房。

circumflex artery
Terminal branch of the left coronary artery irrigating the left ventricle and atrium of the heart.

心前静脉
右心室的小静脉。直接进入右心房。

anterior cardiac veins
Small veins of the right ventricle entering directly into the right atrium.

前室间支
左冠状动脉分支。供应心室和室间隔。

anterior interventricular artery
Branch of the left coronary artery irrigating the ventricles and interventricular septum.

译者注：又叫前降支。

心小静脉
回流心脏右侧的血液的静脉。

small cardiac vein
Vein draining the blood from the right side of the heart.

心大静脉
回流心脏左侧的血液的静脉。

great cardiac vein
Vein draining the blood from the left side of the heart.

胸主动脉
主动脉的第三段。在胸腔降至隔膜，发出位于肋骨之间的多个动脉分支（肋间动脉，肋下动脉）。

thoracic aorta
Third segment of the aorta, descending in the thorax to the diaphragm and giving rise to various arteries located between the ribs (intercostal arteries, subcostal artery).

心尖
心脏的下极。

apex of heart
Lower extremity of the heart.

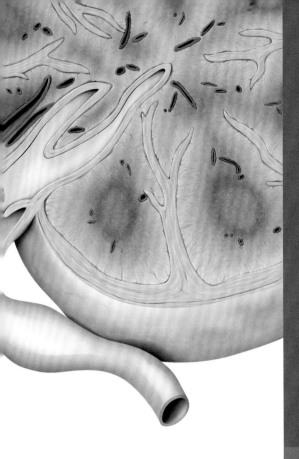

116 淋巴系统器官 organs of the lymphatic system

淋巴系统 Lymphatic system

淋巴系统由淋巴管道和淋巴器官组成，可以产生、储存和激活淋巴细胞。它在免疫和确保组织液回收中起重要作用。淋巴系统与心血管系统紧密相连，它可以将血液容量维持在一个恒定的水平，并使淋巴液回流到血液中。淋巴循环的速度较慢，主要靠压力差运转。

The lymphatic system is composed of lymphatic vessels and lymph organs, which produce, store, and activate lymphocytes. It plays a major role in immunity and ensures tissue drainage. Closely linked to the cardiovascular system, the lymphatic system maintains blood volume at a constant level and returns lymph to the blood. Lymphatic circulation is slow and operates by pressure differential.

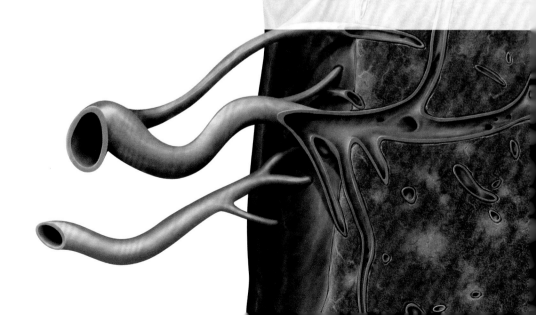

淋巴系统器官

淋巴系统由产生白细胞的初级器官（骨髓和胸腺）与大量产生白细胞和抗体的次级器官（淋巴结、脾脏、扁桃体）组成。

organs of the lymphatic system

The lymphatic system is made up of primary organs (bone marrow and thymus) in which white blood cells are produced and secondary organs (lymph nodes, spleen, tonsils) in which white blood cells and antibodies proliferate.

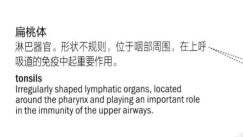

扁桃体
淋巴器官。形状不规则，位于咽部周围，在上呼吸道的免疫中起重要作用。

tonsils
Irregularly shaped lymphatic organs, located around the pharynx and playing an important role in the immunity of the upper airways.

右侧淋巴导管
输送来自身体右上部淋巴液的淋巴管。注入右锁骨下静脉。

right lymphatic duct
Vessel carrying lymph from the upper right section of the body to the right subclavian vein.

胸腺
位于胸骨后面的腺体。某些白细胞在此处成熟。其功能在儿童期尤其活跃。

thymus
Gland located behind the sternum, site of the maturation of certain white blood cells; it is especially active in children.

胸导管
将身体大部分淋巴液输送到左锁骨下静脉的淋巴管。

thoracic duct
Vessel carrying lymph from the largest part of the body to the left subclavian vein.

肠淋巴结
过滤来自肠道淋巴液的淋巴结。

intestinal lymph nodes
Nodes filtering lymph from the intestines.

腘淋巴结
过滤来自膝关节、下肢和足部淋巴液的淋巴结。

popliteal lymph nodes
Nodes filtering lymph from various parts of the knee, leg and foot.

颈部淋巴结
位于颈部的淋巴结。主要过滤来自颈部和部分头部器官和肌肉的淋巴液。

cervical lymph nodes
Nodes found in the neck region, filtering lymph especially from the organs and muscles of the neck and part of the head.

锁骨下静脉
汇集手臂和部分颈部血液的静脉。淋巴液注入其中。

subclavian veins
Veins collecting the blood of the arm and part of the neck; lymph empties into them.

腋淋巴结
位于腋窝的淋巴结。过滤来自上肢和胸腔上部的淋巴液。

axillary lymph nodes
Nodes found in the armpit region, filtering lymph from the upper limbs and upper part of the thorax.

胸部淋巴结
过滤来自胸腔壁和胸部器官淋巴液的淋巴结。

thoracic lymph nodes
Nodes filtering lymph from the walls and organs of the thorax.

脾脏
淋巴器官。位于胃和胰腺之间。它是产生白细胞和抗体的地方，也是血液储存和过滤的地方。

spleen
Lymphatic organ located between the stomach and pancreas; site of the production of white blood cells and antibodies, it is also a place where blood is stored and filtered.

腹股沟淋巴结
主要过滤来自下肢淋巴液的淋巴结。

inguinal lymph nodes
Nodes filtering lymph mainly from the lower limbs.

人体的护卫队 | Army of Protectors

人体大约有500个淋巴结，它们在身体的不同部位形成集群，包括腋窝、颈部、腹股沟和肠道。当发生感染时，白细胞会大量繁殖，淋巴结也会增大。
The body contains about 500 lymph nodes, which form clusters in different parts of the body, including the armpits, the neck, the groin, and the intestines. When there is an infection, the white blood cells multiply and the nodes increase in size.

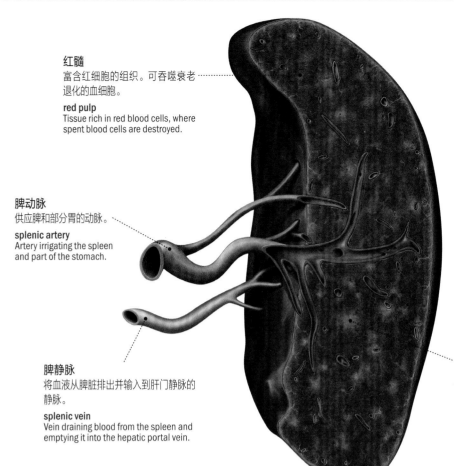

脾脏横截面
脾：淋巴器官。位于胃和胰腺之间，它是产生白细胞和抗体的地方，也是血液储存和过滤的地方。

cross section of spleen
Spleen: lymphatic organ located between the stomach and pancreas; site of the production of white blood cells and antibodies, it is also a place where blood is stored and filtered.

红髓
富含红细胞的组织。可吞噬衰老退化的血细胞。

red pulp
Tissue rich in red blood cells, where spent blood cells are destroyed.

脾动脉
供应脾和部分胃的动脉。

splenic artery
Artery irrigating the spleen and part of the stomach.

脾静脉
将血液从脾脏排出并输入到肝门静脉的静脉。

splenic vein
Vein draining blood from the spleen and emptying it into the hepatic portal vein.

白髓
富含白细胞的组织。可参与免疫反应。

white pulp
Tissue rich in white blood cells that participate in immune reactions.

淋巴管横截面
淋巴管：淋巴液循环的管道。淋巴管形成一个树状网络，从毛细淋巴管排出淋巴液，并单向流往胸导管和右侧淋巴导管。

cross section of a lymphatic vessel
Lymphatic vessel: canal in which lymph circulates; the lymphatic vessels form a treelike network that drains lymph from lymphatic capillaries in one direction toward the thoracic and right lymphatic ducts.

淋巴结横截面
淋巴结：小淋巴器官。沿淋巴管路径分布，过滤和清洁淋巴液。

cross section of a lymph node
Lymph node: small lymphatic organ located along the path of the lymph vessel, filtering and cleaning lymph.

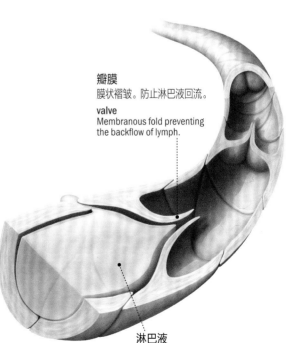

瓣膜
膜状褶皱。防止淋巴液回流。

valve
Membranous fold preventing the backflow of lymph.

淋巴液
半透明的黄色液体。在淋巴管中循环。可确保白细胞能流通至感染部位，从而帮助机体产生免疫作用。

lymph
Translucent clear yellow fluid circulating in the lymphatic vessels; it assists in immunity by ensuring white blood cells circulate to the infected areas.

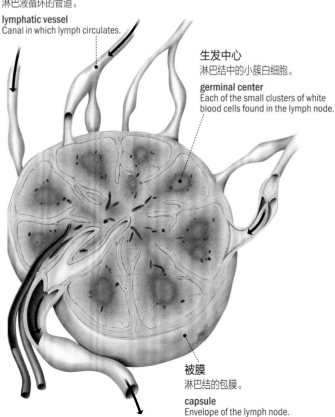

淋巴管
淋巴液循环的管道。

lymphatic vessel
Canal in which lymph circulates.

生发中心
淋巴结中的小簇白细胞。

germinal center
Each of the small clusters of white blood cells found in the lymph node.

被膜
淋巴结的包膜。

capsule
Envelope of the lymph node.

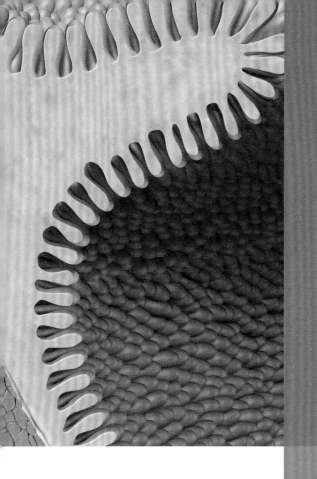

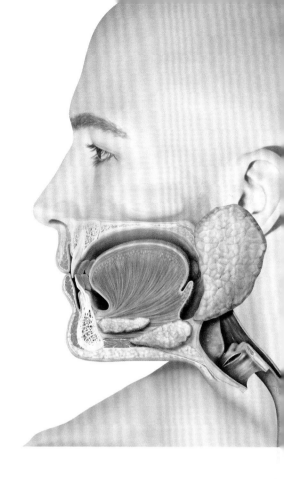

消化系统 Digestive system

消化系统是一组将食物转化为营养物质的器官，即转化为可以被身体直接吸收的成分。因此，它提供了人体生长发育和运转所需的能量和物质。食物通过口腔摄入、咀嚼、唾液消化和吞咽进入消化道，通过机械性消化（收缩）和化学性消化（活性酶）逐渐分解。营养物质、矿物质和水被吸收并在体内循环，而不能被吸收的残渣部分则被排出体外。

The digestive system is the group of organs that transform foods into nutrients—that is, into elements that can be assimilated directly by the body. It thus supplies the energy and raw materials required for the human body to develop and function. Foods are ingested through the mouth, masticated, transformed by saliva, and swallowed. They then enter the digestive tract, where they are gradually broken down by mechanical (contractions) and chemical (enzyme activity) means. Nutrients, minerals, and water are absorbed and circulated throughout the body, while elements that cannot be assimilated are evacuated from the body.

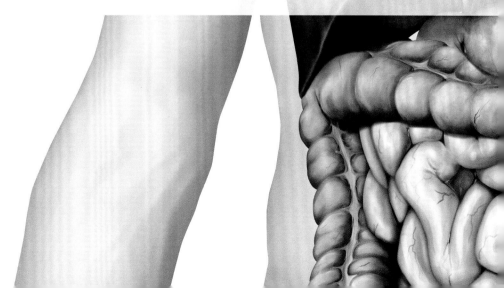

消化系统器官

消化系统由三部分组成：口腔、消化道（食管、胃、肠）和消化腺（唾液腺、肝脏和胰脏）。

organs of the digestive system

The digestive system consists of three parts: the mouth, the digestive tract (esophagus, stomach, intestines) and the appended glands (salivary glands, liver and pancreas).

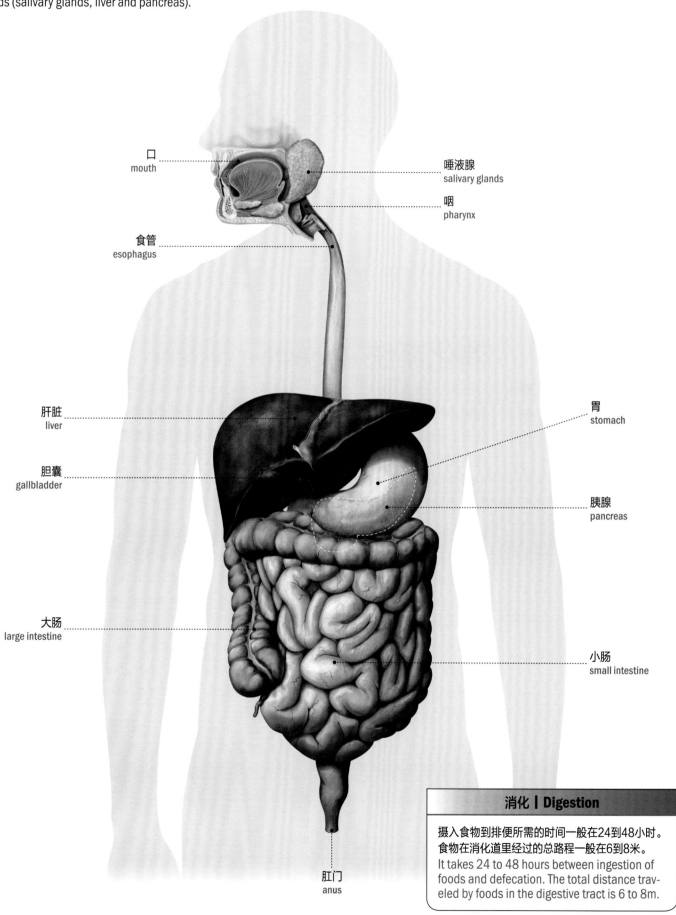

口
mouth

唾液腺
salivary glands

咽
pharynx

食管
esophagus

肝脏
liver

胆囊
gallbladder

胃
stomach

胰腺
pancreas

大肠
large intestine

小肠
small intestine

肛门
anus

消化 ❘ Digestion
摄入食物到排便所需的时间一般在24到48小时。食物在消化道里经过的总路程一般在6到8米。 It takes 24 to 48 hours between ingestion of foods and defecation. The total distance traveled by foods in the digestive tract is 6 to 8m.

消化系统 | DIGESTIVE SYSTEM

口

消化道的起始段。由嘴唇包围着的口腔组成，可以咀嚼消化食物，并在味觉、说话和呼吸中发挥作用。

mouth
Initial part of the digestive tube made up of a cavity (oral cavity) surrounded by lips; it allows the ingestion of food and plays a role in tasting, speaking and breathing.

食管

肌膜通道。位于咽和胃之间，构成上消化道。

esophagus
Muscular membranous channel forming the upper part of the digestive tract, between the pharynx and the stomach.

肝脏

大型腺体。在消化食物和新陈代谢中起重要作用，能分泌胆汁，分解血液中的某些毒素。

liver
Large gland playing an important role in digestion and metabolism; it secretes bile and breaks up certain toxins contained in the blood.

胆囊

小型器官。位于肝脏下面，用来储存和排出胆汁。

gallbladder
Small organ located beneath the liver, serving to store and excrete bile.

大肠

消化道的最后一段。进行最后的消化和废物的排泄。

large intestine
Last segment of the digestive tract, where final digestion and elimination of waste matter take place.

唾液腺

外分泌腺。可分泌唾液。

salivary glands
Exocrine glands secreting saliva.

咽

肌膜通道。既是口腔与食管的结合部，也是鼻腔与喉的结合部，是食物和空气的共用通道。

pharynx
Muscular membranous channel joining the nasal cavities to the larynx as well as the buccal cavity to the esophagus; it serves as a passageway for air and food.

胃

可扩张的囊状消化器官。位于食管和小肠之间，可把食管中的食物转化成浆状物，即食糜。

stomach
Organ of the digestive tract forming an extensible sac between the esophagus and the small intestine; it transforms food from the esophagus into chyme, a thick fluid.

胰腺

狭长型腺体。胰腺位于胃的后部，在消化食物（通过分泌胰液）和调节血糖（通过分泌胰岛素）中起着重要的作用。

pancreas
Elongated gland, located behind the stomach and playing an important role in digestion (secretion of pancreatic juice) and regulation of blood sugar (secretion of insulin).

小肠

消化道的一部分。连接胃和大肠，可部分消化和吸收食物。

small intestine
Channel of the digestive tract joining the stomach to the large intestine, where part of digestion and absorption of food takes place.

肛门

消化道的末端开口。由括约肌控制，排出粪便。

anus
Terminal orifice of the digestive tract, controlled by a sphincter that allows fecal matter to be evacuated.

口 | mouth

口

消化道的起始段。由嘴唇包围着的口腔组成，可以咀嚼消化食物，并在味觉、说话和呼吸中发挥作用。

mouth

Initial part of the digestive tube made up of a cavity (oral cavity) surrounded by lips; it allows the ingestion of food and plays a role in tasting, speaking and breathing.

口外侧观
mouth: external view

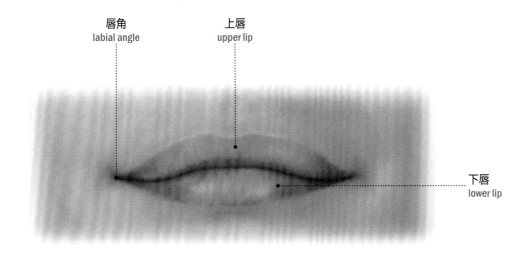

唇角
labial angle

上唇
upper lip

下唇
lower lip

口矢状面
sagittal section of mouth

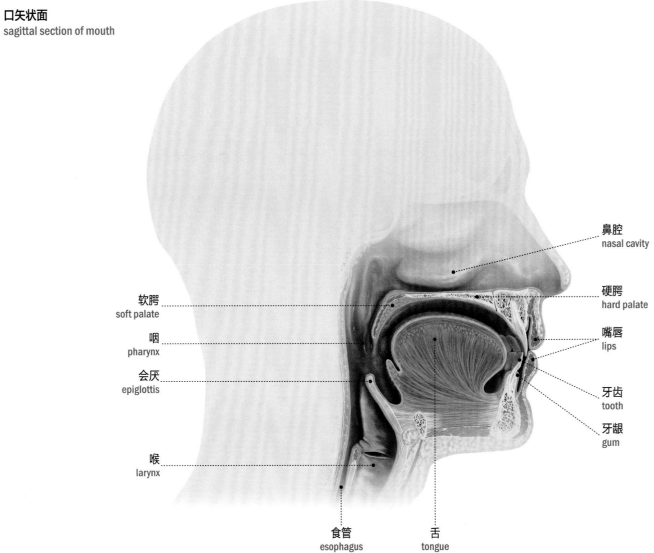

软腭
soft palate

咽
pharynx

会厌
epiglottis

喉
larynx

鼻腔
nasal cavity

硬腭
hard palate

嘴唇
lips

牙齿
tooth

牙龈
gum

食管
esophagus

舌
tongue

唇角
嘴唇的结合部。在口的两侧。

labial angle
Area where the lips join on either side of the mouth.

上唇
构成口上部轮廓的嘴唇。

upper lip
Lip forming the upper contour of the mouth.

下唇
构成口下部轮廓的嘴唇。

lower lip
Lip forming the lower contour of the mouth.

软腭
分隔咽和口腔的肌膜壁。主要作用是辅助进食和发声。

soft palate
Muscular membranous wall separating the pharynx and buccal cavity; it assists especially in ingestion of food and vocalization.

鼻腔
被鼻中隔分隔而成的两个空腔。前开口于鼻孔，后开口于咽部。

nasal cavity
Each of two cavities, separated by the nasal septum, opening in front via the nostrils and in back into the pharynx.

咽
肌膜通道。既是口腔与食管的结合部，也是鼻腔与喉的结合部。是食物和空气的共用通道。

pharynx
Muscular membranous channel joining the nasal cavities to the larynx as well as the buccal cavity to the esophagus; it serves as a passageway for air and food.

硬腭
口腔与鼻腔之间的骨性分隔。硬腭是由软腭延伸而来。

hard palate
Bony separation between the buccal and nasal cavities, extended by the soft palate.

会厌
可活动的软骨瓣。位于喉的上部，吞咽时引导食物进入食管。

epiglottis
Mobile catilaginous lamina located in the upper part of the larynx, directing food to the esophagus at the moment of swallowing.

嘴唇
肉质器官。构成口的前部边界，尤其参与发声功能。

lips
Fleshy organs bounding the front part of the mouth and contributing especially to vocalization.

喉
连接咽和气管的肌性软骨通道，包含声带，具有发声和呼吸功能。

larynx
Muscular cartilaginous channel connecting the pharynx and trachea; it contains the vocal cords and has a vocalizing and respiratory function.

牙齿
发白的坚硬器官。长在上颌骨和下颌骨，用于咀嚼食物。

tooth
Whitish, hard organ borne by the maxilla or mandible and serving to chew food.

食管
肌膜通道。位于咽和胃之间，构成消化道的上部。

esophagus
Muscular membranous channel forming the upper part of the digestive tract, between the pharynx and the stomach.

牙龈
口腔黏膜的较厚部分。富含血管和神经，覆盖上颌骨和下颌骨，包裹牙齿。

gum
Thick part of the buccal mucous membrane rich in blood vessels and nerves, covering the maxilla and mandible and surrounding the teeth.

舌
口腔内的肌性器官。有味觉、咀嚼和说话的功能。

tongue
Muscular organ located in the buccal cavity and involved in tasting, chewing and talking.

牙 | teeth

牙

发白的坚硬器官。根植于上颌骨和下颌骨，用于咀嚼食物。成人的全齿列由32颗牙齿组成。

teeth

Hard, whitish organs implanted in the maxilla and mandible, used for chewing food; full dentition in an adult consists of 32 teeth.

上牙列

上颌骨所萌出的所有牙齿（切牙、尖牙、前磨牙和磨牙）。

upper dentition

All the teeth (incisors, canines, premolars and molars) borne by the maxilla.

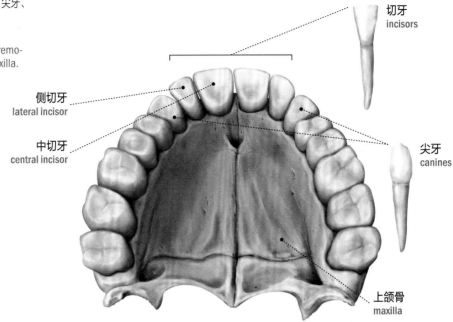

切牙
incisors

侧切牙
lateral incisor

中切牙
central incisor

尖牙
canines

上颌骨
maxilla

下牙列

指下颌骨所萌生的所有牙齿（门牙、尖牙、前磨牙和磨牙）。

lower dentition

All the teeth (incisors, canines, premolars and molars) borne by the mandible.

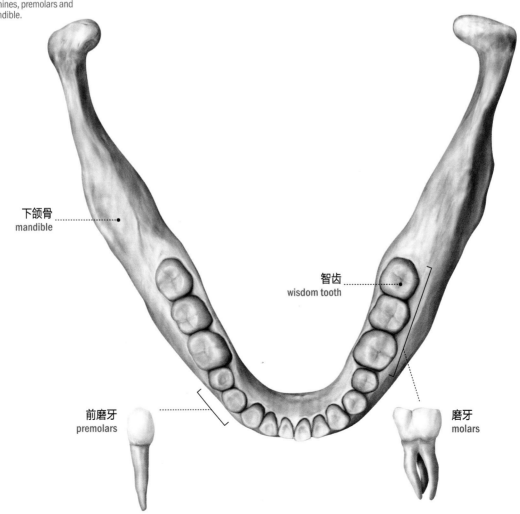

下颌骨
mandible

智齿
wisdom tooth

前磨牙
premolars

磨牙
molars

侧切牙
位于中切牙和尖牙之间的切牙。

lateral incisor
Incisor located between the central incisor and the canine.

切牙
位于上颌骨和下颌骨前部的扁平牙齿（共有8颗），边缘较锋利，方便咬入食物。

incisors
Flat teeth (8) located in the front of the maxilla and mandible, having a cutting edge that allows them to bite into food.

中切牙
位于牙齿前部的切牙。

central incisor
Incisor located in the front section of teeth.

尖牙
位于切牙和前磨牙之间的牙齿（共有4颗），有尖顶，能够咬穿和撕碎食物。

canines
Teeth (4) located between the incisors and the premolars, having a pointed crown that is able to pierce and tear food.

上颌骨
组成软腭、部分硬腭、眼眶和鼻腔的成对骨。

maxilla
Paired bone forming the upper jaw, part of the hard palate, orbits and nasal cavity.

下颌骨
不成对的骨。组成下颌，与颞骨形成关节，以便于咀嚼。

mandible
Unpaired bone forming the lower jaw, articulating with the temporal bones to allow chewing.

智齿
牙弓的最后一颗磨牙，一般出现在18到30岁之间，但有些人没有长出。

wisdom tooth
Last molar of the dental arch, appearing generally between the ages of 18 and 30 but missing in some people.

前磨牙
位于尖牙和磨牙之间的牙齿（总共8颗），它们与磨牙作用相同，但是作用较小。

premolars
Teeth (8) located between the canines and molars; they play the same role as molars but are smaller.

磨牙
位于上颌骨和下颌骨后部的牙齿（总共12颗），磨牙体型较大，有两个或三个牙根及一个扁平的牙冠，用来研磨食物。

molars
Teeth (12) located at the back of the maxilla and mandible; large in size with two or three roots, they have a flat crown that allows them to grind food.

磨牙截面

牙齿由两部分组成：牙冠-从牙龈中露出的部分，便于咀嚼，牙根-植入上下颌骨的部分。牙根可有一个或多个。

section of a molar

A tooth is made up of two parts: the crown that emerges from the gum and ensures chewing, and one or more roots that are inserted into the bone.

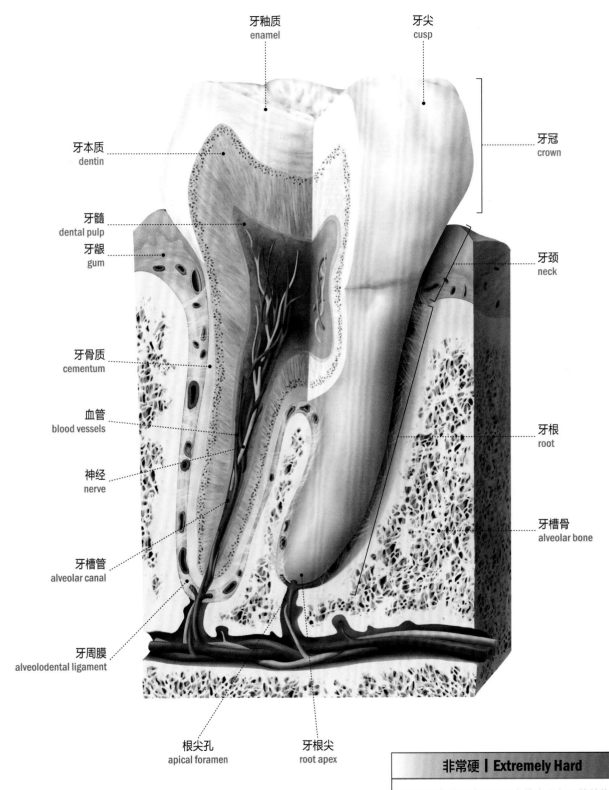

牙釉质
enamel

牙尖
cusp

牙本质
dentin

牙髓
dental pulp

牙龈
gum

牙骨质
cementum

血管
blood vessels

神经
nerve

牙槽管
alveolar canal

牙周膜
alveolodental ligament

牙冠
crown

牙颈
neck

牙根
root

牙槽骨
alveolar bone

根尖孔
apical foramen

牙根尖
root apex

非常硬 | Extremely Hard

覆盖牙齿的牙釉质层是人体内最坚硬的结构。牙本质的硬度稍软一点，但仍差不多像骨头一样坚硬。

The layer of enamel that covers the teeth is the hardest structure in the human body. Dentin is slightly softer, but still almost as hard as a bone.

牙釉质
保护牙冠和部分牙齿颈部的极其坚硬的矿物质。

enamel
Extremely resistant mineral substance protecting the crown and part of the neck of the tooth.

牙本质
构成牙齿主体的硬钙化组织。

dentin
Very hard calcified tissue forming the largest part of the tooth.

牙髓
牙齿内部的结缔组织。包含毛细血管、淋巴管和神经。

dental pulp
Connective tissue forming the middle part of the tooth and containing the blood capillaries, lymphatic vessels and nerves.

牙龈
口腔黏膜的较厚部分。富含血管和神经，覆盖上颌骨和下颌骨，包裹牙齿。

gum
Thick part of the buccal mucous membrane rich in blood vessels and nerves, covering the maxilla and mandible and surrounding the teeth.

牙骨质
薄层类似于骨的组织，覆盖于牙齿根部。

cementum
Thin layer of tissue, similar to bone tissue, covering the root of the tooth.

血管
血液循环的通道。由动脉、毛细血管和静脉组成。

blood vessels
Canals through which blood circulates; there are arteries, capillaries and veins.

神经
由神经纤维组成的长索。在中枢神经系统和身体其他部位之间传递感觉或运动信息。

nerve
Long cord formed of nerve fibers, carrying sensory or motor messages between the central nervous system and the rest of the body.

牙槽管
位于牙根中心的通道。允许毛细血管、淋巴管和神经通过。

alveolar canal
Channel located at the centre of the root of the tooth, allowing the passage of blood capillaries, lymphatic vessels and nerves.

牙周膜
将牙齿固定在牙槽骨中的韧带。

alveolodental ligament
Ligament anchoring the tooth in the alveolar bone.

根尖孔
每根牙根根部的孔。允许毛细血管、淋巴管和神经通过牙槽管。

apical foramen
Aperture at the base of each root of the tooth, allowing the passage of blood capillaries, lymphatic vessels and nerves toward the alveolar canal.

牙尖
前磨牙和磨牙上侧的牙釉质形成的尖端，方便研磨食物。

cusp
Point formed by the enamel on the upper side of premolars and molars, allowing them to grind food.

牙冠
牙齿的外部，覆盖着牙釉质，确保咀嚼食物。

crown
Outer part of the tooth, covered in enamel, ensuring chewing.

牙颈
牙齿缩窄部分。在牙冠和牙根之间，由牙龈包裹。

neck
Constricted part of the tooth, between the crown and roots, surrounded by the gum.

牙根
嵌入上下颌骨中的牙齿部分。由牙周膜固定。

root
Part of the tooth embedded in the bone, where it is held in place by the alveolodental ligament.

牙槽骨
上颌骨下缘、下颌骨的上缘。包含齿槽（牙槽），牙齿镶嵌其中。

alveolar bone
Superficial part of the maxilla and mandible, containing sockets (dental alveoli) in which the teeth are inserted.

牙根尖
牙根的末端。

root apex
Extremity of the root.

消化道

消化道是输送和消化食物的所有中空器官（食管、胃、肠），它们彼此相连形成一条6至8米长的管道，上端始于咽喉，下端终于肛门。

digestive tract

All the hollow organs (esophagus, stomach, intestines) allowing food to be transported and digested; they succeed one another to form a conduit 6 to 8m long that joins the pharynx to the anus.

胃
stomach

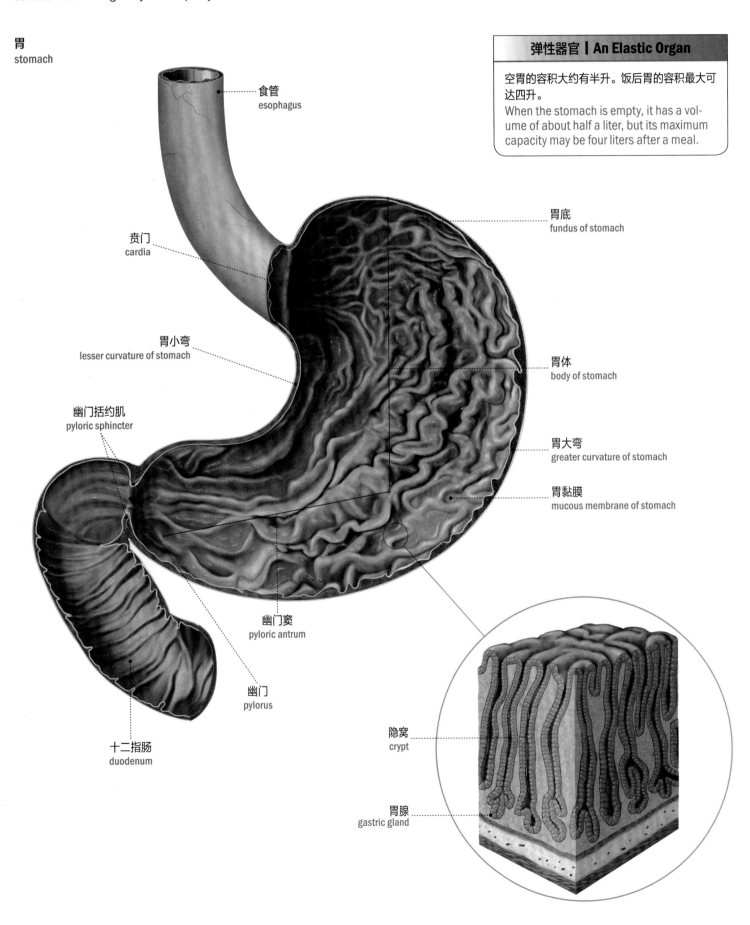

弹性器官 | An Elastic Organ

空胃的容积大约有半升。饭后胃的容积最大可达四升。

When the stomach is empty, it has a volume of about half a liter, but its maximum capacity may be four liters after a meal.

食管
esophagus

贲门
cardia

胃小弯
lesser curvature of stomach

幽门括约肌
pyloric sphincter

幽门窦
pyloric antrum

幽门
pylorus

十二指肠
duodenum

胃底
fundus of stomach

胃体
body of stomach

胃大弯
greater curvature of stomach

胃黏膜
mucous membrane of stomach

隐窝
crypt

胃腺
gastric gland

胃
可扩张的囊状消化器官。位于食管和小肠之间，把来自食管的食物消化成浆状物，即食糜。

stomach
Organ of the digestive tract forming an extensible sac between the esophagus and the small intestine; it transforms food from the esophagus into chyme, a thick fluid.

食管
肌膜通道。位于咽和胃之间，构成消化道的上部。

esophagus
Muscular membranous channel forming the upper part of the digestive tract, between the pharynx and the stomach.

胃底
胃的上部。

fundus of stomach
Upper part of the stomach.

贲门
胃的上开口。与食管相连。

cardia
Upper orifice of the stomach connecting with the esophagus.

胃体
胃的主要部分，位于胃底和幽门之间。

body of stomach
Main part of the stomach contained between the fundus and pylorus.

胃小弯
胃的右缘。

lesser curvature of stomach
Right border of the stomaach.

胃大弯
胃的左缘。

greater curvature of stomach
Left border of the stomach.

幽门括约肌
环状肌肉。用于闭合幽门，其舒张时，可让食物进入十二指肠。

pyloric sphincter
Ring-like muscle closing the pylorus; when released, it allows the passage of food into the duodenum.

胃黏膜
被覆胃内壁的黏膜。可产生多种分泌物（黏液、胃液）。

mucous membrane of stomach
Mucous membrane covering the inner side of the stomach and producing various secretions (mucus, gastric juice).

十二指肠
小肠的起始段。与胃相连，接收来自肝脏和胰腺的分泌物。

duodenum
Initial segment of the small intestine, connecting with the stomach and receiving the secretions of the liver and pancreas.

隐窝
胃黏膜内形成的深褶。胃黏膜的隐窝可容纳四到五个胃腺。

crypt
Deep fold formed inside a mucous membrane; crypts of the gastric mucous membrane can house four or five gastric glands.

幽门窦
胃的最底部。

pyloric antrum
Lower part of the stomach.

胃腺
外分泌腺。位于隐窝后面，生产胃液。胃液酸性很强，有助于消化食物。

gastric gland
Exocrine gland located at the back of a crypt and producing gastric juice, a highly acidic liquid aiding in food digestion.

幽门
胃的下开口。与十二指肠相连。

pylorus
Lower orifice of the stomach connecting with the duodenum.

小肠

连接胃和大肠的消化道。可以部分消化和吸收食物。

small intestine

Channel of the digestive tract joining the stomach to the large intestine, where part of digestion and absorption of food takes place.

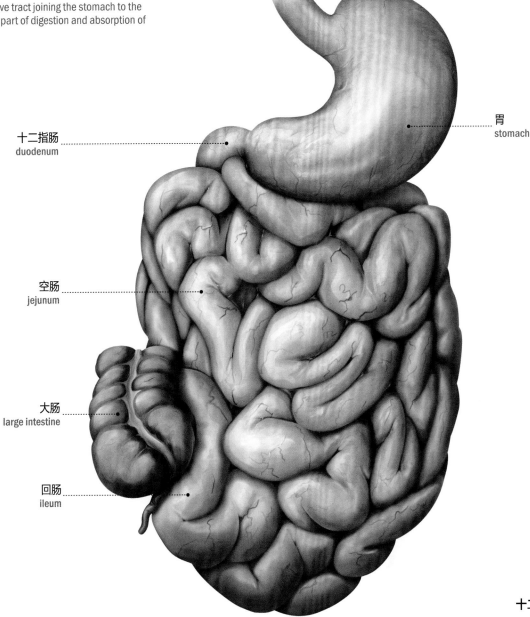

十二指肠
duodenum

胃
stomach

空肠
jejunum

大肠
large intestine

回肠
ileum

十二指肠截面

section of duodenum

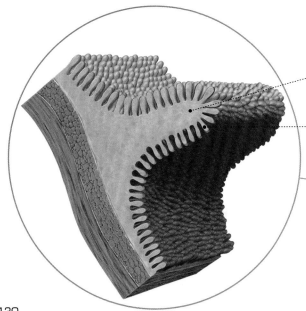

环状褶
circular fold

肠绒毛
intestinal villus

小肠黏膜
mucous membrane of small intestine

十二指肠

小肠的起始段。与胃相连，接收来自肝脏和胰腺的分泌物。

duodenum

Initial segment of the small intestine, connecting with the stomach and receiving secretions from the liver and pancreas.

胃

可扩张的囊状消化器官。位于食管和小肠之间。把来自食管的食物消化成浆状物，即食糜。

stomach

Organ of the digestive tract forming an extensible sac between the esophagus and the small intestine; it transforms food from the esophagus into chyme, a thick fluid.

空肠

小肠的第二段。位于十二指肠和回肠之间，是人体吸收营养的主要部位。

jejunum

Second segment of the small intestine between the duodenum and ileum, ensuring the major part of nutrient absorption.

大肠

消化道的最后一段。这里进行最后消化和废物排泄。

large intestine

Last segment of the digestive tract, in which final digestion and waste elimination take place.

回肠

小肠的末段。与大肠相连。

ileum

Terminal segment of the small intestine, connecting with the large intestine.

环状褶

小肠黏膜形成的大的环状皱襞。

circular fold

Large circular fold formed by the mucous membrane of the small intestine.

小肠黏膜

小肠内壁的黏膜。产生帮助吸收营养的肠液。

mucous membrane of small intestine

Mucous membrane lining the inner side of the small intestine and producing the intestinal juice, a liquid that assists in nutrient absorption.

肠绒毛

小肠黏膜的皱褶。可以增大小肠的吸收面积。

intestinal villus

Fold of the mucous membrane of the small intestine allowing the absorptive surface to increase.

大肠
消化道的最后一段。这里进行最后的消化和废物排泄。

large intestine
Last segment of the digestive tract, where final digestion and elimination of waste matter take place.

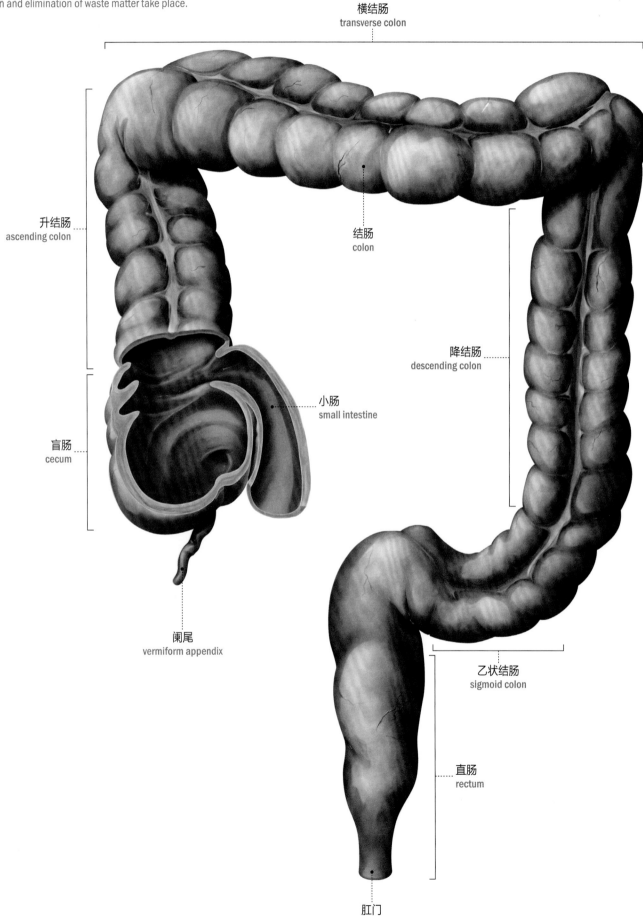

横结肠
transverse colon

升结肠
ascending colon

结肠
colon

降结肠
descending colon

盲肠
cecum

小肠
small intestine

阑尾
vermiform appendix

乙状结肠
sigmoid colon

直肠
rectum

肛门
anus

横结肠

结肠的水平段。位于升结肠和降结肠之间。

transverse colon
Horizontal segment of the colon between the ascending colon and the descending colon.

结肠

位于盲肠和直肠之间的大肠的一部分，分为四段。

colon
Part of the large intestine located between the cecum and rectum and divided into four segments.

升结肠

结肠的起始部。在腹部的右侧，升结肠从食物残渣中吸收水分。

ascending colon
Initial segment of the colon, in the right part of the abdomen, where water from food residue is absorbed.

降结肠

结肠的第三段。位于腹部左侧，代谢废物在排泄之前暂存于此。

descending colon
Third segment of the colon, in the left part of the abdomen, where waste matter is stored before being excreted.

盲肠

大肠的起始部。与小肠相连。

cecum
Initial part of the large intestine, connecting with the small intestine.

小肠

消化道的一部分。连接胃和大肠，可部分消化和吸收食物。

small intestine
Channel of the digestive tract joining the stomach to the large intestine, where part of digestion and absorption of food takes place.

阑尾

位于盲肠末端的大肠的延伸部分，内有大量淋巴结。

vermiform appendix
Outgrowth of the large intestine located at the extremity of the cecum and containing numerous lymph nodes.

乙状结肠

结肠的末端，可以将代谢废物运送到直肠。

sigmoid colon
Terminal segment of the colon, carrying waste matter toward the rectum.

直肠

大肠的末端。与肛门的外部相连，可使粪便通过。

rectum
Terminal segment of the large intestine, connecting with the outside of the anus and allowing defecation.

隐藏的生物 | Hidden Fauna

结肠中约有400多种不同的细菌，数量多达几十亿个。这些细菌的功能各有不同，有的能生产维生素、有的能消化特定物质，有的能摧毁病原体。

The colon houses billions of bacteria of about 400 different species. These bacteria perform various functions related to production of vitamins, digestion of some substances, and destruction of pathogens.

肛门

消化道的末端开口。由括约肌控制，可使粪便排出。

anus
Terminal orifice of the digestive tract, controlled by a sphincter that allows fecal matter to be evacuated.

胰腺 | pancreas

消化系统 | DIGESTIVE SYSTEM

胰腺
狭长型腺体。在消化食物（通过分泌胰液）和调节血糖（通过分泌胰岛素）中起着重要的作用。

pancreas
Elongated gland playing an important role in digestion (secretion of pancreatic juices) and in control of blood sugar (secretion of insulin).

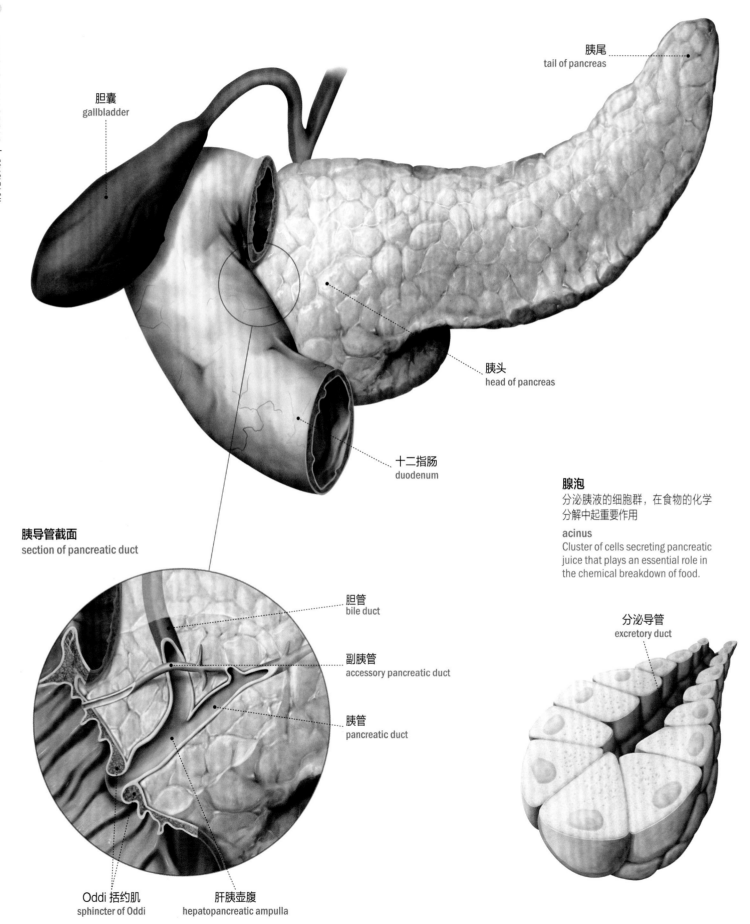

胰尾
tail of pancreas

胆囊
gallbladder

胰头
head of pancreas

十二指肠
duodenum

胰导管截面
section of pancreatic duct

胆管
bile duct

副胰管
accessory pancreatic duct

胰管
pancreatic duct

Oddi 括约肌
sphincter of Oddi

肝胰壶腹
hepatopancreatic ampulla

腺泡
分泌胰液的细胞群，在食物的化学分解中起重要作用

acinus
Cluster of cells secreting pancreatic juice that plays an essential role in the chemical breakdown of food.

分泌导管
excretory duct

胆囊
位于肝脏下面的小器官。用来储存和排出胆汁。
gallbladder
Small organ located beneath the liver, serving to store and excrete bile.

胰头
胰腺的一部分，紧贴十二指肠。
head of pancreas
Part of the pancreas lodged against the duodenum.

胰尾
胰腺的左端。
tail of pancreas
Left extremity of the pancreas.

十二指肠
小肠的起始段。与胃相连，接收肝脏和胰腺的分泌物。
duodenum
Initial segment of the small intestine, connecting with the stomach and receiving secretions from the liver and pancreas.

胆管
将胆汁输送到十二指肠的管道。
bile duct
Canal serving to carry bile to the duodenum.

分泌导管
导管。收集胰液，并输送至胰管。
excretory duct
Canal collecting pancreatic juice and carrying it to the pancreatic duct.

副胰管
胰管分支。由肝胰壶腹进入十二指肠的上游。
accessory pancreatic duct
Branch of the pancreatic duct discharging into the duodenum upstream from the hepatopancreatic ampulla.

胰管
收集胰腺产生的胰液并将其排送至肝胰壶腹的管道。
pancreatic duct
Canal collecting pancreatic juice produced by the pancreas and emptying it into the hepatopancreatic ampulla.

Oddi 括约肌
位于肝胰壶腹开口周围的环状括约肌。调节流向十二指肠的分泌物。
sphincter of Oddi
Ring-like muscle surrounding the aperture of the hepatopancreatic ampulla; it regulates the passage of secretions toward the duodenum.

肝胰壶腹
开口于十二指肠的管道。由胰管与胆管的结合部形成。
hepatopancreatic ampulla
Canal resulting from the juncture of the pancreatic duct and the bile duct, discharging into the duodenum.

肝脏 | liver

肝脏
大型腺体。在食物消化和新陈代谢中起重要作用，能分泌胆汁，可分解血液中的某些毒素。
liver
Large gland playing an important role in digestion and metabolism; it secretes bile and breaks up certain toxins contained in the blood.

肝脏前面观
liver: anterior view

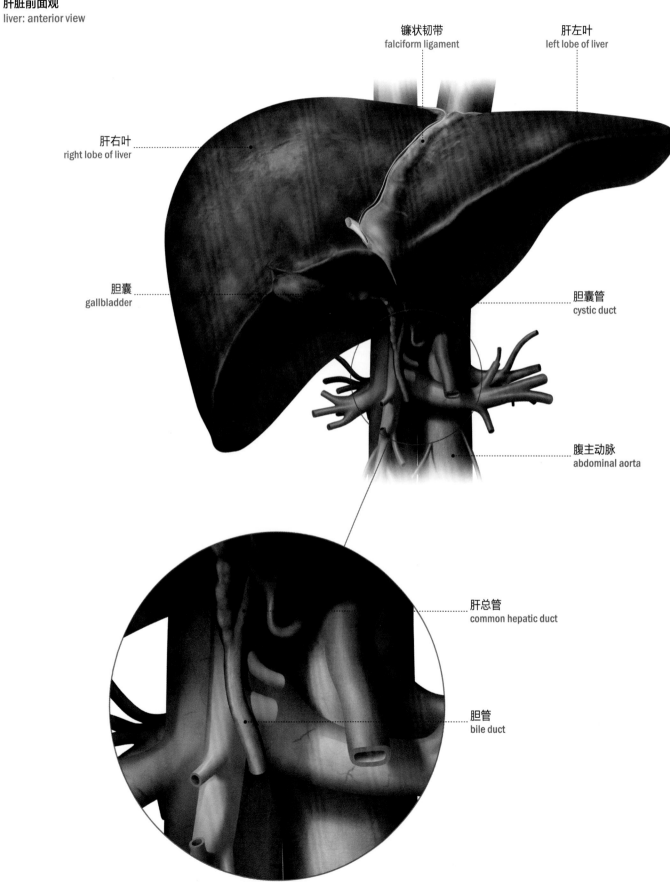

镰状韧带
falciform ligament

肝左叶
left lobe of liver

肝右叶
right lobe of liver

胆囊
gallbladder

胆囊管
cystic duct

腹主动脉
abdominal aorta

肝总管
common hepatic duct

胆管
bile duct

镰状韧带
分隔肝左右叶的膜状物。
falciform ligament
Membrane separating the right and left lobes of the liver.

左肝叶
肝脏的一部分。位于镰状韧带左侧。
left lobe of liver
Part of the liver located to the left of the falciform ligament.

右肝叶
肝脏的主要部分。位于镰状韧带的右侧。
right lobe of liver
Main part of the liver, located to the right of the falciform ligament.

胆囊管
连接胆囊和胆管的管道。胆汁在其中循环。
cystic duct
Canal connecting the biliary vesicle to the bile duct, in which bile circulates.

胆囊
位于肝脏下面的小器官。用来储存和排泄胆汁。
gallbladder
Small organ located beneath the liver, serving to store and excrete bile.

腹主动脉
主动脉的第四段。也是最后一段。向下进入腹腔并形成多个分支，主要通向肾脏、胰腺和结肠。
abdominal aorta
Fourth and last segment of the aorta, passing down into the abdominal cavity and giving rise to various arteries leading especially toward the kidneys, pancreas and colon.

肝总管
肝脏排出胆汁的通道。与胆囊管相连，形成胆管。
common hepatic duct
Canal through which the liver excretes bile, connecting with the cystic duct to form the bile duct.

胆管
由胆囊管和肝总管连接而成的管道。将胆汁输送到十二指肠。
bile duct
Canal formed by the joining of the cystic duct and the common hepatic duct, carrying bile to the duodenum.

庞大的器官 | A Voluminous Organ

肝脏是人体的最大内脏器官。平均重量约为1.5千克。也是进行化学转化最多的器官。
The liver, which reaches an average weight of about 1.5kg, is the largest internal organ in the human body. It is also the organ that performs the largest number of chemical transformations.

消化系统 | DIGESTIVE SYSTEM

肝门脉系统

肝门脉系统包括把血液从消化道输送到肝脏的所有静脉；它帮助肝脏处理血液并保留消化产生的营养物质。

hepatic portal system
All the veins draining blood from the digestive tract to the liver; it allows the liver to process the blood and retain many substances produced by digestion.

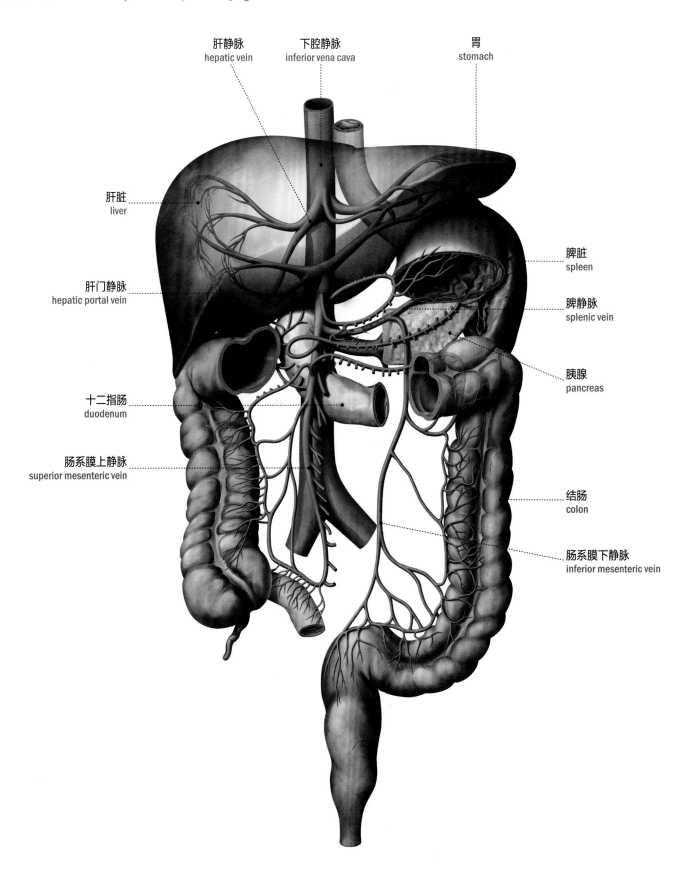

肝静脉
hepatic vein

下腔静脉
inferior vena cava

胃
stomach

肝脏
liver

脾脏
spleen

肝门静脉
hepatic portal vein

脾静脉
splenic vein

胰腺
pancreas

十二指肠
duodenum

肠系膜上静脉
superior mesenteric vein

结肠
colon

肠系膜下静脉
inferior mesenteric vein

肝静脉

将肝脏过滤后的血液输送到下腔静脉的血管。

hepatic vein
Vein draining the blood filtered by the liver and emptying it into the inferior vena cava.

肝脏

大型腺体。在食物消化和新陈代谢中起重要作用，能分泌胆汁，可分解血液中的某些毒素。

liver
Large gland playing an important role in digestion and metabolism; it secretes bile and breaks up certain toxins contained in the blood.

肝门静脉

将血液从肠、胃、胰腺和脾脏输送到肝脏的血管。

hepatic portal vein
Vein carrying blood from the intestines, stomach, pancreas and spleen to the liver.

十二指肠

小肠的起始段。与胃相连，接收肝脏和胰腺的分泌物。

duodenum
Initial segment of the small intestine, connecting with the stomach and receiving the secretions of the liver and pancreas.

肠系膜上静脉

将小肠和升结肠的血液输送到肝门静脉的血管。

superior mesenteric vein
Vein carrying the blood of the small intestine and ascending colon to the hepatic portal vein.

下腔静脉

将身体下部（横膈膜下方）收集来的乏氧血输送至右心房的静脉。

inferior vena cava
Vein carrying deoxygenated blood from the lower part of the body (below the diaphragm) to the right atrium of the heart.

胃

可扩张的囊状消化器官。位于食管和小肠之间，把来自食管的食物消化成浆状物，即食糜。

stomach
Organ of the digestive tract forming an extensible sac between the esophagus and the small intestine; it transforms food from the esophagus into chyme, a thick fluid.

脾脏

淋巴器官。位于胃和胰腺之间。可以制造白细胞和抗体，同时也可以储存和过滤血液。

spleen
Lymphatic organ located between the stomach and pancreas; site of the production of white blood cells and antibodies, it is also a place where blood is stored and filtered.

脾静脉

将血液从脾脏和结肠输送到肝门静脉的血管。

splenic vein
Vein carrying blood from the spleen and colon to the hepatic portal vein.

胰腺

狭长型腺体。在消化食物（通过分泌胰液）和调节血糖（通过分泌胰岛素）中起着重要的作用。

pancreas
Elongated gland playing an important role in digestion (secretion of pancreatic juices) and in control of blood sugar (secretion of insulin).

结肠

大肠的一部分。位于盲肠和直肠之间。

colon
Part of the large intestine between the cecum and the rectum.

肠系膜下静脉

将降结肠和乙状结肠的血液输送到脾静脉的血管。

inferior mesenteric vein
Vein carrying the blood of the descending colon and sigmoid colon to the splenic vein.

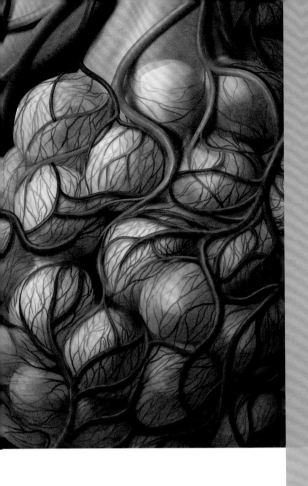

呼吸系统 Respiratory system

呼吸系统由持续参与空气和血液交换的多个器官组成。这些器官能不间断地供给人体所需的氧气，同时排除人体产生的二氧化碳。空气由胸廓的运动吸入，由上呼吸道（气管和支气管）到达肺，在肺泡进行气体交换。除呼吸功能外，呼吸系统在说话和嗅觉方面也起着至关重要的作用。

The respiratory system is the group of organs that are involved in a constant exchange between air and blood in order to supply the body with the oxygen it needs and eliminate the carbon dioxide that it produces. Air, inhaled due to movement of the thoracic cage, flows through the upper respiratory tract, the trachea and bronchia, and reaches the alveoli in the lungs, where gas exchanges take place. Aside from breathing, the respiratory system plays an essential role in speech and the sense of smell.

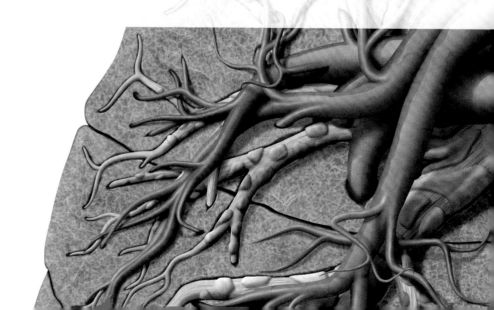

呼吸系统器官

呼吸系统由上呼吸道、气管和肺组成。

organs of the respiratory system

The respiratory system is made up of the upper respiratory tract, trachea and lungs.

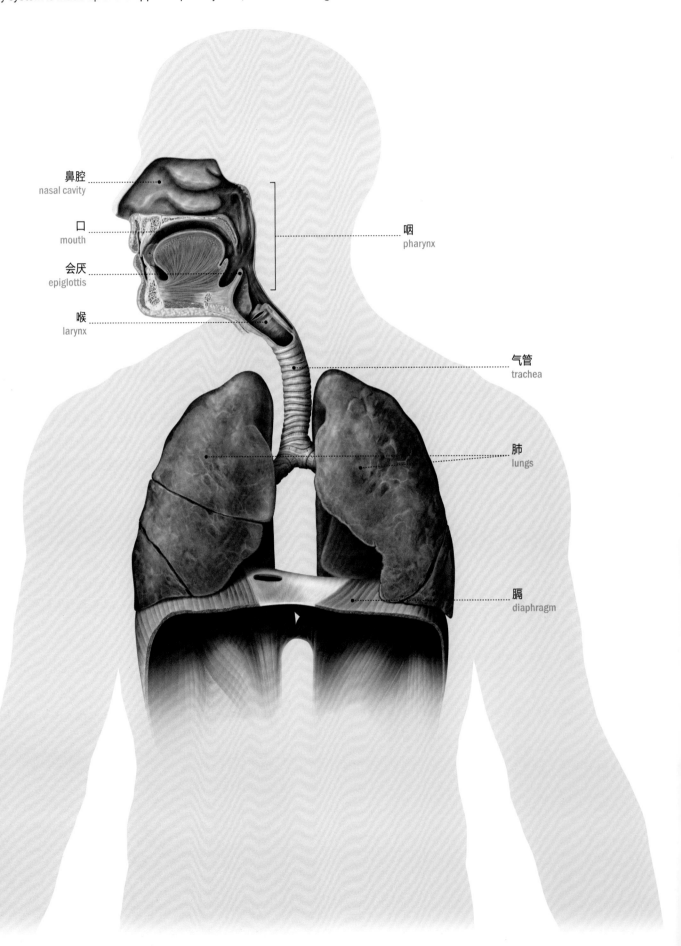

鼻腔
nasal cavity

口
mouth

会厌
epiglottis

喉
larynx

咽
pharynx

气管
trachea

肺
lungs

膈
diaphragm

鼻腔

由鼻中隔分隔而成的两个空腔。前开口通于鼻孔，后开口连于咽部。

nasal cavity
Each of two cavities, separated by the nasal septum, opening in front via the nostrils and in back into the pharynx.

咽

肌膜通道。既是口腔与食管的结合部，也是鼻腔与喉的结合部，是食物和空气的共用通道。

pharynx
Muscular membranous channel joining the nasal cavities to the larynx as well as the buccal cavity to the esophagus; it serves as a passageway for air and food.

口

消化道的起始段。由嘴唇包围着的空腔（口腔）组成，它可以咀嚼、消化食物，并在味觉、说话和呼吸中发挥作用。

mouth
Initial part of the digestive tube made up of a cavity (oral cavity) surrounded by lips; it allows the ingestion of food and plays a role in tasting, speaking and breathing.

气管

肌性软骨通道。位于喉和支气管之间，可使空气通过。

trachea
Muscular cartilaginous channel allowing air to pass between the larynx and bronchi.

会厌

软骨瓣。位于喉的上部，可活动，吞咽时引导食物进入食管。

epiglottis
Mobile catilaginous lamina located in the upper part of the larynx, directing food to the esophagus at the moment of swallowing.

肺

呼吸器官。由弹性组织构成，负责空气和血液间的气体交换。

lungs
Organs of the respiratory system made of elastic tissues and responsible for the exchange of gases between the air and the blood.

喉

肌性软骨通道。连接咽和气管，包含声带，具有发声和呼吸功能。

larynx
Muscular cartilaginous channel connecting the pharynx and trachea; it contains the vocal cords and has a vocalizing and respiratory function.

膈

分隔胸腔和腹腔的肌肉，其收缩会增加胸廓和肺的容积。

diaphragm
Muscle separating the thorax from the abdomen; its contraction increases the volume of the thoracic cage and lungs.

空气运动 | Air Movements

某些特定的自发性运动，可以从呼吸道排出异物颗粒。 咳嗽能清除支气管、气管或喉咙的异物。打喷嚏会在鼻腔产生强烈气流，速度可高达约150千米/小时。

Certain movements occur spontaneously to dislodge undesirable particles from the respiratory tract. Coughing clears the bronchial tubes, the trachea, or the throat, while sneezing produces a strong air current in the nasal cavity, with an estimated speed of 150km/h.

上呼吸道

使空气从气管进入肺的器官。由鼻、口、咽、喉组成。

upper respiratory tract
Organ allowing air to pass from the trachea to the lungs; it consists of the nose, mouth, pharynx and larynx.

鼻子

面部中间的突出部分。有两个孔（鼻孔），具有嗅觉和呼吸功能。

nose
Protrusion in midsection of the face, with two orifices (nostrils), having an olfactory and respiratory function.

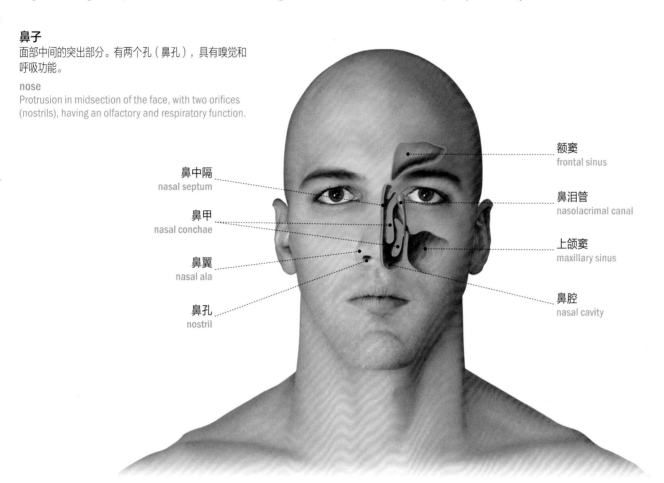

鼻中隔
nasal septum

鼻甲
nasal conchae

鼻翼
nasal ala

鼻孔
nostril

额窦
frontal sinus

鼻泪管
nasolacrimal canal

上颌窦
maxillary sinus

鼻腔
nasal cavity

鼻旁窦

面部的骨性空腔，通过狭窄的孔与鼻腔相通，使头骨重量减轻并产生黏液。

paranasal sinuses
Cavities in the bones of the face, connecting with the nasal cavities through narrow orifices; they reduce the weight of the bones of the head and produce mucus.

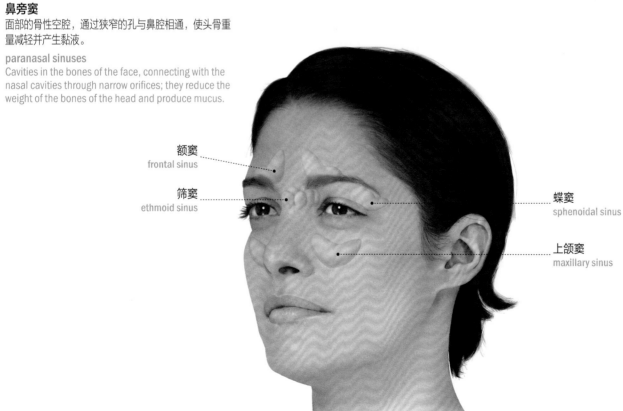

额窦
frontal sinus

筛窦
ethmoid sinus

蝶窦
sphenoidal sinus

上颌窦
maxillary sinus

鼻中隔

软骨薄壁。分隔两个鼻腔。

nasal septum
Thin cartilaginous wall separating the two nasal cavities.

额窦

额骨的空腔。与鼻腔相通，加热吸入的空气。

frontal sinus
Cavity in the frontal bone, connecting with the nasal cavities and warming inhaled air.

鼻甲

鼻腔壁的骨性延伸。可预热和湿润吸入的空气。

nasal conchae
Bony extensions of the wall of the nasal cavities, serving to warm and humidify inhaled air.

鼻泪管

使泪液排入鼻腔的通道。

nasolacrimal canal
Channel through which tears are evacuated toward the nasal cavities.

鼻翼

鼻下部的软骨部分。由其围成鼻孔。

nasal ala
Lower cartilaginous part of the nose, bordering the nostril.

上颌窦

上颌骨内充气的空腔。与鼻腔相通。

maxillary sinus
Air-filled cavity in the maxilla, connecting with the nasal cavities.

鼻孔

鼻的开孔。空气由此进入鼻腔。

nostril
Orifice of the nose through which air enters the nasal cavities.

鼻腔

由鼻中隔分隔而成的两个空腔。前开口通于鼻孔，后开口连于咽部。

nasal cavity
Each of two cavities, separated by the nasal septum, opening in front via the nostrils and in back into the pharynx.

额窦

额骨的空腔。与鼻腔相通，加热吸入的空气。

frontal sinus
Cavity in the frontal bone, connecting with the nasal cavities and warming inhaled air.

蝶窦

蝶骨的空腔。与鼻腔相通，加热吸入的空气。

sphenoidal sinus
Cavity in the sphenoid bone, connecting with the nasal cavities and warming inhaled air.

筛窦

筛骨的空腔。与鼻腔相通。

ethmoid sinus
Cavity in the ethmoid bone, connecting with the nasal cavities.

上颌窦

上颌骨内充气的空腔。与鼻腔相通。

maxillary sinus
Air-filled cavity in the maxilla, connecting with the nasal cavities.

上呼吸道矢状面
sagittal section of upper respiratory tract

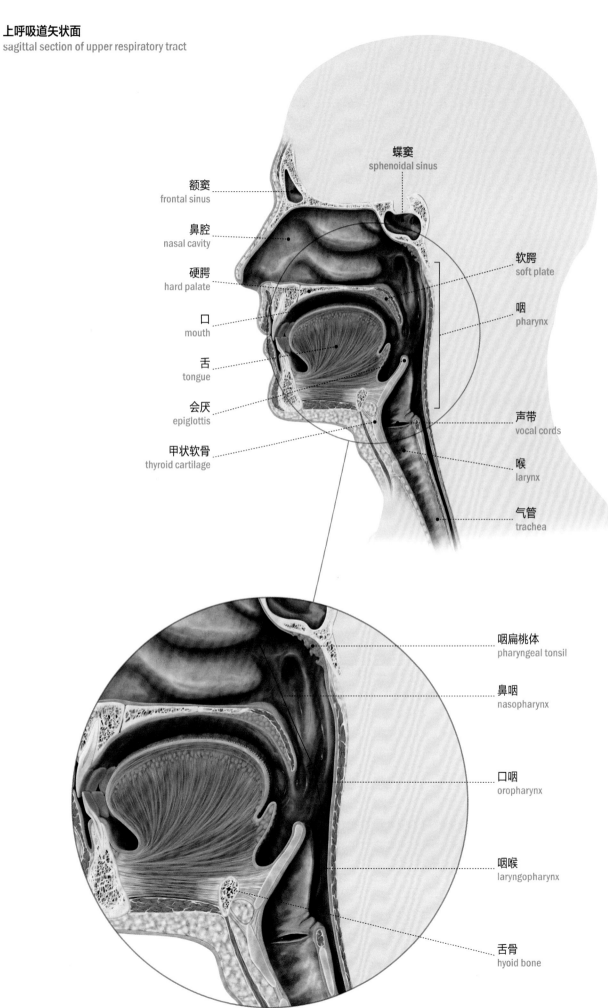

蝶窦
sphenoidal sinus

额窦
frontal sinus

鼻腔
nasal cavity

硬腭
hard palate

口
mouth

舌
tongue

会厌
epiglottis

甲状软骨
thyroid cartilage

软腭
soft plate

咽
pharynx

声带
vocal cords

喉
larynx

气管
trachea

咽扁桃体
pharyngeal tonsil

鼻咽
nasopharynx

口咽
oropharynx

咽喉
laryngopharynx

舌骨
hyoid bone

额窦

额骨的空腔。与鼻腔相通，加热吸入的空气。

frontal sinus
Cavity in the frontal bone, connecting with the nasal cavities and warming inhaled air.

鼻腔

鼻腔被鼻中隔分为两个腔。向前借鼻孔通外界，向后通向咽部。

nasal cavity
Each of two cavities, separated by the nasal septum and opening in front through the nostrils and in back into the nasopharynx.

硬腭

骨性分隔。由软腭延伸而来，使口腔与鼻腔分隔。

hard palate
Bony separation between the buccal and nasal cavities, extended by the soft palate.

口

消化道的起始段。由嘴唇包围着的空腔（即口腔）组成，可以咀嚼消化食物，并在味觉、说话和呼吸中发挥作用。

mouth
Initial part of the digestive tube made up of a cavity (oral cavity) surrounded by lips; it allows the ingestion of food and plays a role in tasting, speaking and breathing.

舌

口腔内的肌性器官。有味觉、咀嚼和说话的功能。

tongue
Muscular organ located in the buccal cavity and involved in tasting, chewing and talking.

会厌

软骨瓣。位于喉的上部，可活动，吞咽时引导食物进入食管。

epiglottis
Mobile catilaginous lamina located in the upper part of the larynx, directing food to the esophagus at the moment of swallowing.

甲状软骨

由两片侧向的薄层结缔组织结构构成。其结合部会在男性的咽喉前部形成一处明显的突起，即喉结。

thyroid cartilage
Connective tissue structure formed of two lateral laminae whose juncture, on the front part of the larynx, forms a highly visible protrusion in men (Adam's apple).

蝶窦

蝶骨的空腔。与鼻腔相通，加热吸入的空气。

sphenoidal sinus
Cavity in the sphenoid bone, connecting with the nasal cavities and warming inhaled air.

软腭

肌膜分隔。使鼻咽部和口腔分隔，尤在摄入食物和发声方面起作用。

soft plate
Muscular membranous wall separating the nasopharynx and buccal cavity; it assists especially in food ingestion and vocalization.

咽

肌膜通道。既是口腔与食管的结合部，也是鼻腔与喉的结合部，是食物和空气的共用通道。

pharynx
Muscular membranous channel joining the nasal cavities to the larynx as well as the buccal cavity to the esophagus; it serves as a passageway for air and food.

声带

长带状肌肉组织。附着在甲状软骨和杓状软骨上，震动可以发出声音。

vocal cords
Long bands of muscle tissue attached to the thyroid and arytenoid cartilages; their vibration allows sounds to be produced.

喉

肌性软骨通道。连接咽和气管，内含声带，具有发声和呼吸功能。

larynx
Muscular cartilaginous channel connecting the pharynx and trachea; it contains the vocal cords and has a vocalizing and respiratory function.

气管

肌性软骨通道。位于喉和支气管之间，可使空气通过。

trachea
Muscular cartilaginous channel allowing air to pass between the larynx and bronchi.

咽扁桃体

鼻咽部的淋巴器官。可以过滤空气中的病原体。

pharyngeal tonsil
Lymphoid organ located in the nasopharynx, filtering pathogens from the air.

鼻咽

咽的上部。与鼻腔相连。

nasopharynx
Upper part of the pharynx connecting with the nasal cavities.

口咽

咽的中部。与口腔相连。

oropharynx
Median part of the pharynx connecting with the buccal cavity.

咽喉

咽的下部。与喉和食管相连。

laryngopharynx
Lower part of the pharynx connecting with the larynx and esophagus.

舌骨

支撑喉的骨骼。提供舌、咽和喉等多处的肌肉止点。

hyoid bone
Bone supporting the larynx and serving as an insertion for various muscles of the tongue, pharynx and larynx.

肺 | lungs

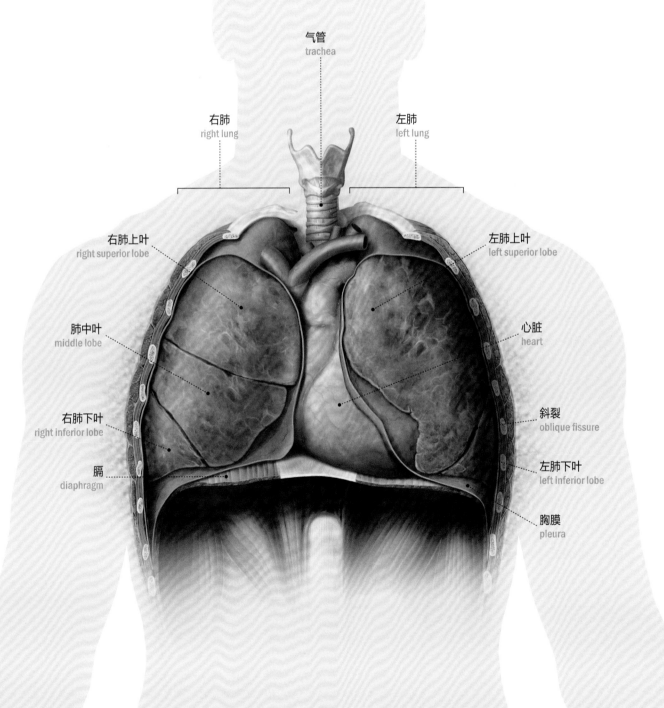

肺
由弹性组织构成的呼吸器官，负责空气和血液间的气体交换。

lungs
Organs of the respiratory system made of elastic tissues and responsible for the exchange of gases between the air and the blood.

呼吸 | Respiration
成人的静态呼吸频率为15次/分钟，即每天呼吸超过21 000次。每次吸气，都会将半升的含氧空气通过呼吸道吸入到肺。

An adult at rest breathes about 15times a minute, or more than 21,000 times per day. With each inhalation, a half-liter of air loaded with oxygen passes through the respiratory tract to the lungs.

气管
trachea

右肺
right lung

左肺
left lung

右肺上叶
right superior lobe

左肺上叶
left superior lobe

肺中叶
middle lobe

心脏
heart

右肺下叶
right inferior lobe

斜裂
oblique fissure

膈
diaphragm

左肺下叶
left inferior lobe

胸膜
pleura

气管
肌性软骨通道。位于喉和支气管之间，可使空气通过。
trachea
Muscular cartilaginous channel allowing air to pass between the larynx and bronchi.

左肺
呼吸器官。分两叶，左肺动脉血在此释放二氧化碳，吸收氧气。
left lung
Respiratory organ divided into two lobes, in which blood from the left pulmonary artery is freed of carbon dioxide and enriched with oxygen.

右肺
呼吸器官。分三叶，右肺动脉血在此释放二氧化碳，吸收氧气。
right lung
Respiratory organ divided into three lobes, in which blood from the right pulmonary artery is freed of carbon dioxide and enriched with oxygen.

左肺上叶
左肺上部。通过斜裂与下叶分开。
left superior lobe
Upper part of the left lung, separated from the inferior lobe by an oblique fissure.

右肺上叶
右肺上部。通过水平裂与下叶和中叶分开。
right superior lobe
Upper part of the right lung, separated from the inferior lobe and middle lobe by a horizontal fissure.

心脏
肌性器官。分成四个腔，通过自主并有规律的收缩，推动血液在全身循环。
heart
Muscular organ divided into four chambers whose autonomous rhythmic contractions cause blood to circulate throughout the body.

肺中叶
右肺的一部分。通过斜裂与上叶和中叶分开。
middle lobe
Part of the right lung, separated from the superior lobe and inferior lobe by an oblique fissure.

斜裂
分隔肺叶的裂隙。
oblique fissure
Fissure separating the lobes of the lung.

右肺下叶
右肺下部。通过斜裂与上叶和中叶分开。
right inferior lobe
Lower part of the right lung, separated from the superior lobe and middle lobe by an oblique fissure.

左肺下叶
左肺下部。通过斜裂与上叶分开。
left inferior lobe
Lower part of the left lung, separated from the superior lobe by an oblique fissure.

膈
分隔胸腔和腹腔的肌肉。其收缩会增加胸廓和肺的容量。
diaphragm
Muscle separating the thorax from the abdomen; its contraction increases the volume of the thoracic cage and lungs.

胸膜
包绕肺的弹性膜。由胸膜腔的两层膜组成。
pleura
Elastic membrane surrounding each lung and composed of two layers bounding the pleural cavity.

支气管树

可使空气进入肺的所有气道。包含两条主支气
管，主支气管再继续分支，最后变成细支气管。

bronchial tree
All the airways allowing air to reach the lungs;
it contains two main bronchi whose successive
divisions lead to the bronchioles.

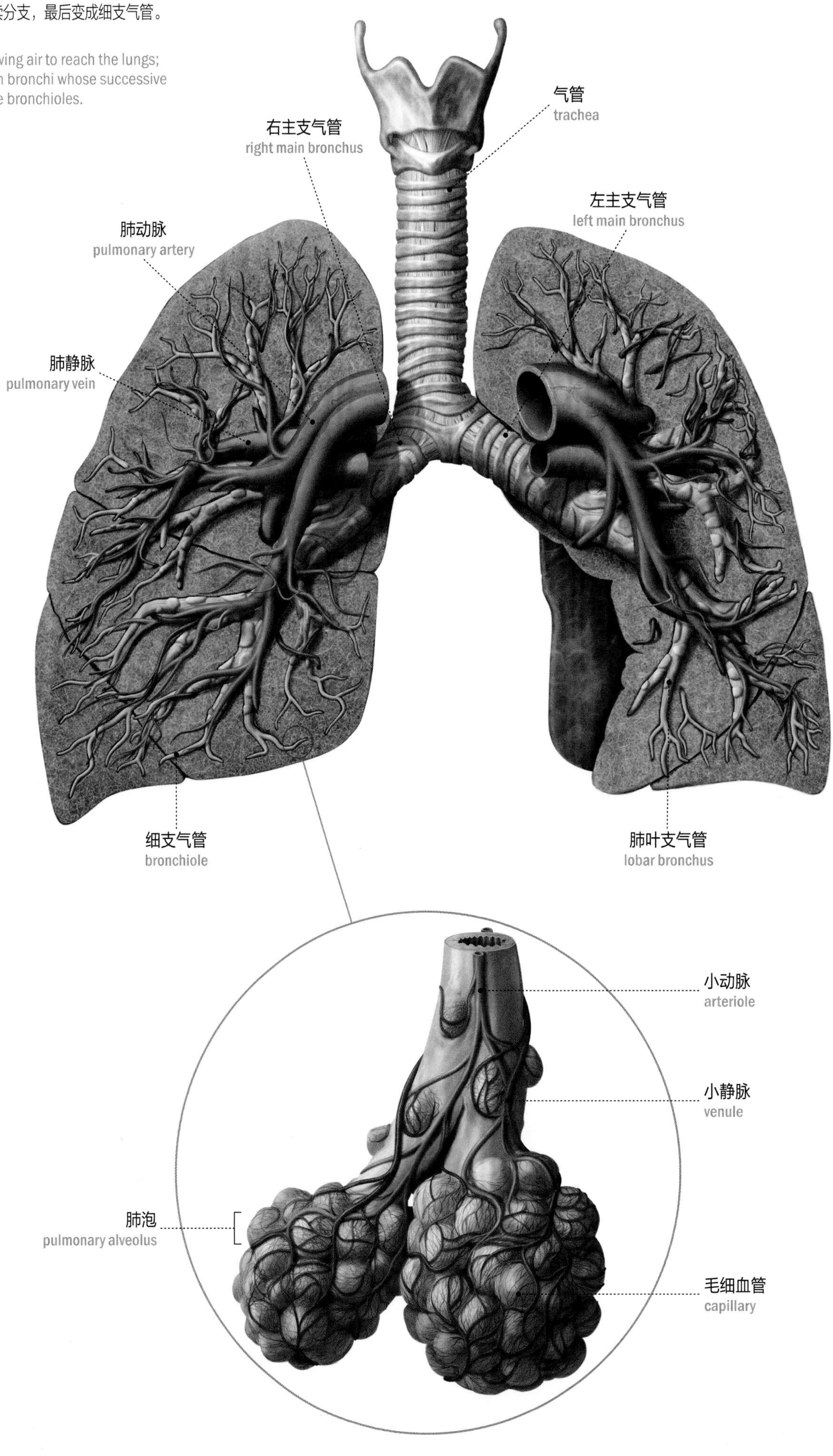

气管
trachea

右主支气管
right main bronchus

左主支气管
left main bronchus

肺动脉
pulmonary artery

肺静脉
pulmonary vein

细支气管
bronchiole

肺叶支气管
lobar bronchus

小动脉
arteriole

小静脉
venule

肺泡
pulmonary alveolus

毛细血管
capillary

右主支气管
从气管分出的支气管。使空气进出右肺。

right main bronchus
Bronchus emanating from the trachea, allowing air to enter and exit the right lung.

肺动脉
肺动脉干的分支。将乏氧血输送到肺。

pulmonary artery
Branch of the pulmonary trunk carrying deoxygenated blood to the lungs.

肺静脉
将富氧血从肺输送到左心房的静脉。

pulmonary vein
Vein carrying oxygenated blood from the lungs to the left chamber of the heart.

细支气管
支气管树最狭窄的部分。止于肺泡。

bronchiole
The narrowest subdivision of the bronchial tree, ending in the pulmonary alveoli.

肺泡
小囊泡。位于细支气管的末端，成簇排列，肺泡由一层薄壁（呼吸膜）包裹，可与毛细血管进行气体交换。

pulmonary alveolus
Small cavity located at the extremity of the bronchioles; grouped in clusters, the alveoli are surrounded by a thin wall that allows gaseous exchanges with the capillaries.

气管
肌性软骨通道。位于喉和支气管之间，可使空气通过。

trachea
Muscular cartilaginous channel allowing air to pass between the larynx and bronchi.

左主支气管
从气管分出的支气管。使空气进出左肺。

left main bronchus
Bronchus emanating from the trachea, allowing air to enter and exit the left lung.

肺叶支气管
主支气管的所有众多分支。为肺叶提供空气。

lobar bronchus
Each of very numerous twigs of the main bronchus supplying air to the pulmonary lobe.

小动脉
肺动脉末端的细小分支。终于毛细血管网。

arteriole
Fine terminal branch of the pulmonary artery, ending in a capillary network.

小静脉
位于毛细血管的延伸处的细小静脉。与肺静脉相连。

venule
Small-sized vein located in the extension of a capillary and joining up with the pulmonary vein.

毛细血管
微细血管。保障小动脉和小静脉间的血液循环，其管壁允许血液与毛细血管的外界进行物质交换。

capillary
Tiny blood vessel ensuring blood circulation between an arteriole and a venule; its wall allows exchanges between the blood and exterior of the capillary.

气管
肌性软骨通道。位于喉和支气管之间，可使空气通过。

trachea
Muscular cartilaginous channel allowing air to pass between the larynx and bronchi.

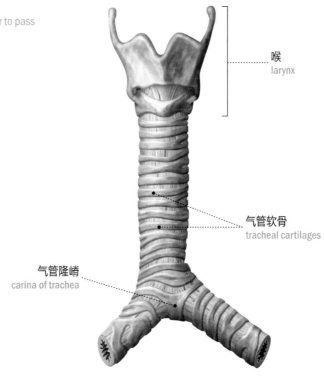

喉
larynx

气管软骨
tracheal cartilages

气管隆嵴
carina of trachea

胸膜
两肺周围的弹性膜。分为脏壁两层，构成胸膜腔。

pleura
Elastic membrane surrounding each lung and composed of two sheets bounding the pleural cavity.

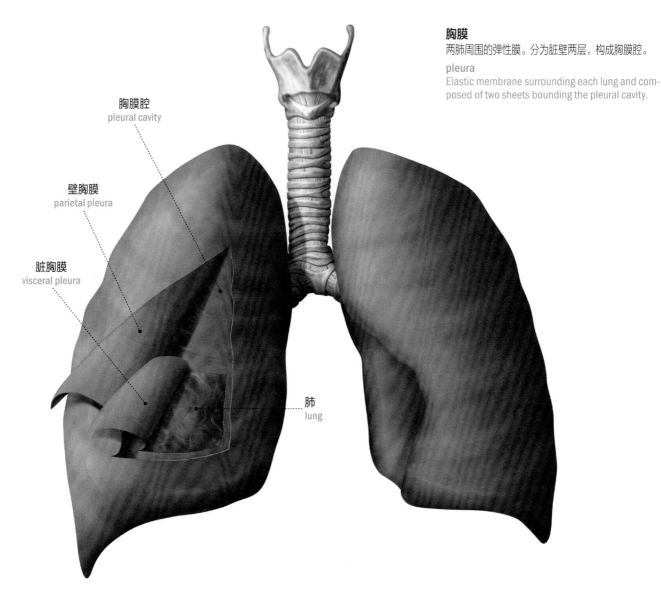

胸膜腔
pleural cavity

壁胸膜
parietal pleura

脏胸膜
visceral pleura

肺
lung

气体交换的场所 | Area for Exchange

肺有超过3亿个肺泡。肺泡的总面积相当于一个网球场。

The lungs house more than 300 million alveoli. The total area of the pulmonary alveoli is the size of a tennis court.

喉
肌性软骨通道。连接咽和气管，内含声带，有发声和呼吸功能。

larynx
Muscular cartilaginous channel connecting the pharynx and trachea; it contains the vocal cords and has a vocalizing and respiratory function.

气管隆嵴
气管的下部分。分成两条支气管。

carina of trachea
Lower part of the trachea dividing into two bronchi.

气管软骨
软骨环。构成气管壁，有16~20个。作用是支撑气管，保持通畅。

tracheal cartilages
Cartilaginous rings (16 to 20) contained in the wall of the trachea, allowing it to remain open.

胸膜腔
胸膜的壁层与脏层之间的空隙。内含胸膜液，有润滑作用，利于胸膜之间的滑动，有助于完成呼吸运动。

pleural cavity
Cavity between the parietal and visceral layers of the pleura; it contains a lubricating fluid (pleural fluid) allowing them to slide, thus contributing to respiration.

肺
呼吸器官。由弹性组织构成，负责空气和血液之间的气体交换。

lung
Organ of the respiratory tract formed of extensible tissue and responsible for gaseous exchanges between air and blood.

壁胸膜
胸膜的外层。与胸廓和横膈膜相接。

parietal pleura
Outer layer of the pleura, in contact with the thoracic cage and diaphragm.

脏胸膜
胸膜的内层。与肺紧贴。

visceral pleura
Inner layer of the pleura, in contact with the lung.

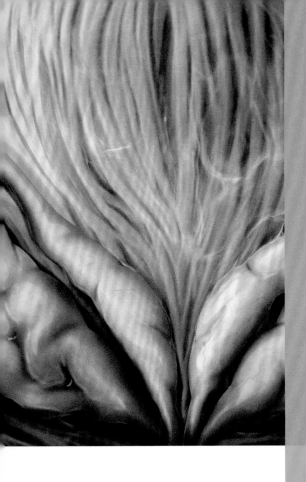

泌尿系统 Urinary system

泌尿系统由一组生成、运输和储存尿液，然后将其排出体外的器官组成。男性和女性的上尿路器官（肾脏和输尿管）相同，而下尿路（膀胱和尿道）不同。泌尿系统与肾脏的血液循环系统相连，肾脏负责过滤血液。过滤后的产物（尿液）会暂存在膀胱，之后排出体外。

The urinary system is the group of organs that make, transport, and store urine, and then evacuate it from the body. The organs of the upper urinary tract (kidneys and ureters) are identical in both sexes, while the bladder and urethra, which form the lower urinary tract, are different in men and women. The urinary system is connected to the blood circulation system in the kidneys, which filter the blood. The product of this filtration, urine, is stored temporarily in the bladder before it is eliminated.

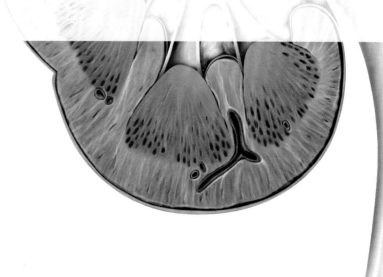

泌尿系统器官

泌尿系统的上部分由输尿管和肾脏组成，而下部分由膀胱和尿道组成。

organs of the urinary system

The upper part of the urinary system consists of the ureters and kidneys, while the lower urinary tract is made up of the bladder and urethra.

男性前面观
man: anterior view

肾脏
位于腹部的两个器官。主要功能是过滤血液，形成尿液。

kidney
Each of two organs located in the abdomen whose main function is to produce urine by filtering the blood.

膀胱
中空器官。暂时收集肾脏产生的尿液，在排尿时通过尿道排空。

urinary bladder
Hollow organ in which urine produced in the kidneys temporarily collects; it empties through the urethra during urination.

肾上腺
内分泌腺。位于肾脏上方，可分泌多种激素，其中有的参与应激反应，有的参与水平衡。

suprarenal gland
Endocrine gland located above the kidney; some of the hormones it secretes are involved in the stress response while others act on water retention.

输尿管
肌膜通道。共有两条，将尿液从肾脏输送到膀胱。

ureter
Each of two muscular membranous channels carrying urine from the kidneys to the bladder.

男性尿道
通道。起始于膀胱底，穿过前列腺，沿阴茎走行，止于尿道口，可排尿和射精。

male urethra
Channel originating at the base of the bladder, crossing the prostate and running along the penis to the urethral orifice; it allows urination and ejaculation.

女性前面观
woman: anterior view

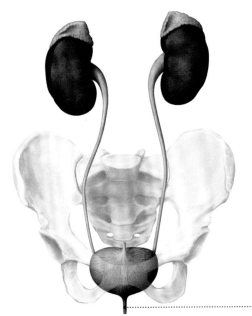

尿量 | Liquid Quantities

泌尿系统在人的一生中平均能产生4.5万升尿液，足以充满一个直径5米左右的游泳池。

The human urinary system produces an average of 45,000 liters of urine over a lifetime – enough to fill a swimming pool about 5 meters in diameter.

女性尿道
通道。起始于膀胱底，排尿时尿液由此通过，其出口（外口）位于阴蒂和阴道口之间。

female urethra
Channel originating at the base of the bladder and through which urine flows during urination; its exit hole (meatus) is located between the vaginal opening and the clitoris.

膀胱
中空器官。暂时收集肾脏产生的尿液，在排尿时通过尿道排空。
urinary bladder
Hollow organ in which urine produced in the kidneys temporarily collects; it empties through the urethra during urination.

膀胱前剖面
frontal section of urinary bladder

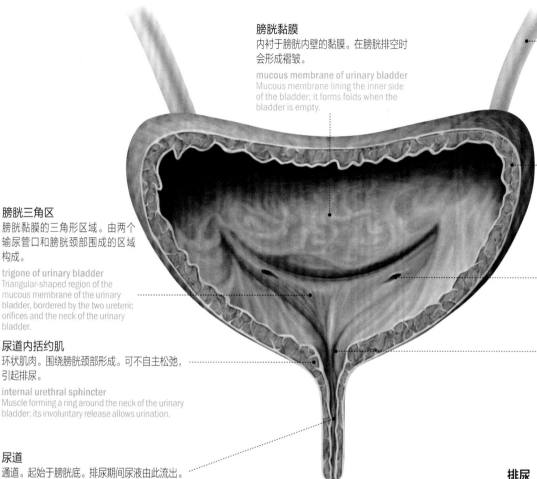

膀胱黏膜
内衬于膀胱内壁的黏膜。在膀胱排空时会形成褶皱。

mucous membrane of urinary bladder
Mucous membrane lining the inner side of the bladder; it forms folds when the bladder is empty.

输尿管
肌膜通道。共有两条，将尿液从肾脏输送到膀胱。

ureter
Each of two muscular membranous channels carrying urine from the kidneys to the bladder.

逼尿肌
平滑肌。构成膀胱壁的主要部分。

detrusor muscle
Smooth muscle forming the essential part of the bladder wall.

膀胱三角区
膀胱黏膜的三角形区域。由两个输尿管口和膀胱颈部围成的区域构成。

trigone of urinary bladder
Triangular-shaped region of the mucous membrane of the urinary bladder, bordered by the two ureteric orifices and the neck of the urinary bladder.

输尿管口
输尿管与膀胱相连的开口。

ureteric orifice
Opening through which the ureter connects with the bladder.

尿道内括约肌
环状肌肉。围绕膀胱颈部形成。可不自主松弛，引起排尿。

internal urethral sphincter
Muscle forming a ring around the neck of the urinary bladder; its involuntary release allows urination.

膀胱颈
膀胱的下端。与尿道相连。

neck of urinary bladder
Lower extremity of the bladder connecting with the urethra.

尿道
通道。起始于膀胱底。排尿期间尿液由此流出。

urethra
Channel originating at the base of the bladder and through which urine flows during urination.

排尿
通过尿道排空膀胱中尿液的过程。

urination
Voiding through the urethra of urine stored in the bladder.

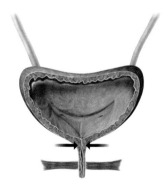

储尿
来自肾脏的尿液通过输尿管排入膀胱。尿道的内括约肌收缩，使通往尿道的入口关闭。

filling
Urine from the kidneys empties into the bladder through the ureters; the internal urethral sphincter contracts to close the entrance to the urethra.

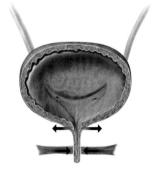

憋尿
当膀胱半充盈时，尿道的内括约肌会松弛。可以通过尿道的外括约肌自主收缩来憋尿。

retention
When the bladder is half full, the internal urethral sphincter releases; urine can be held by the voluntary contraction of an external urethral sphincter.

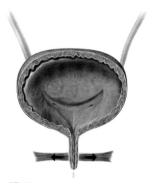

排尿
通过尿道排空膀胱中尿液的过程。

urination
Voiding through the urethra of urine stored in the bladder.

肾脏

位于腹部的两个器官。主要功能是过滤血液。

kidney

Each of two organs located in the abdomen whose main function is to filter the blood.

肾脏前面观

kidneys: anterior view

下腔静脉
将身体下部（横膈下方）收集来的乏氧血液输送至右心房的静脉。

inferior vena cava
Vein carrying deoxygenated blood from the lower part of the body (below the diaphragm) to the right atrium of the heart.

肾上腺
内分泌腺。位于肾脏上方，可分泌多种激素，其中有的参与应激反应，有的参与水分平衡。

suprarenal gland
Endocrine gland located above the kidney; certain hormones that it secretes assist in the stress mechanism, while others act on water retention.

腹主动脉
主动脉的第四段。也是最后一段。向下进入腹腔并形成多个分支，分别通向肾脏、胰腺和结肠。

abdominal aorta
Fourth and last segment of the aorta, passing down into the abdominal cavity and giving rise to various arteries leading especially toward the kidneys, pancreas and colon.

肾动脉
腹主动脉分支。供血给肾脏。

renal artery
Branch of the abdominal aorta irrigating the kidney.

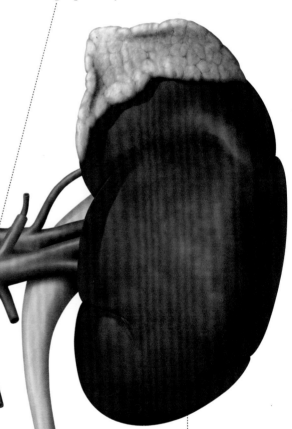

右肾
位于肝脏下面的器官。主要功能是过滤血液。

right kidney
Organ located beneath the liver; its main function is to filter the blood.

肾静脉
接收肾脏过滤后的血液并送回下腔静脉。

renal vein
Vein receiving blood filtered by the kidney and carrying it to the inferior vena cava.

左肾
位于脾脏下面的器官。主要功能是过滤血液。

left kidney
Organ located beneath the spleen; its main function is to filter the blood.

输尿管
肌膜通道。共有两条，将尿液从肾脏输送到膀胱。

ureter
Each of two muscular membranous channels carrying urine from the kidneys to the bladder.

肾脏前剖面
frontal section of right kidney

肾皮质
肾脏的一部分。内含肾小球。
renal cortex
Part of the kidney containing the glomeruli.

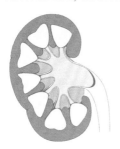

肾髓质
肾脏的中间部分。由肾锥体组成。
renal medulla
Middle part of the kidney, made up of renal pyramids.

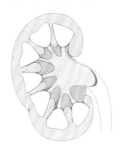

纤维囊
肾脏的包膜。
fibrous capsule
Membrane enveloping the kidney.

肾锥体
肾髓质的基本成分。由许多集合管组成。
renal pyramid
Element of the renal medulla consisting of a grouping of many collecting ducts.

肾盏
腔体。收集来自集合管的尿液。
renal calix
Cavity collecting urine coming from the collecting ducts.

肾盂
漏斗形腔体。由肾盏集合形成，末端在输尿管内。
renal pelvis
Funnel-shaped cavity formed by the union of calices and ending in the ureter.

肾柱
肾皮质的延伸。在两个肾锥体之间。
renal column
Extension of the renal cortex between two pyramids.

输尿管
肌膜通道。共有两条，将尿液从肾脏输送到膀胱。
ureter
Each of two muscular membranous channels carrying urine from the kidneys to the bladder.

肾单位
肾脏的功能单位。尿液在此产生，由两种主要成分组成：肾小球和肾小管。
nephron
Functional unit of the kidney where urine is produced; it is formed of two main elements: the glomerulus and the renal tubule.

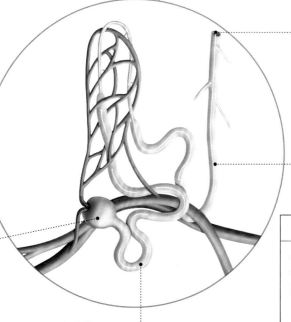

尿液
由肾脏血液过滤产生的液体。储存在膀胱并在排尿时排出，尿液的95%都是水，其中溶解着多种代谢产物。
urine
Liquid resulting from the filtration of blood in the kidneys, stored in the bladder and evacuated during urination; urine is made up of 95% water in which various substances left over from metabolism are dissolved.

集合管
管道。收集肾单位产生的尿液并将其输送到肾盏。
collecting duct
Duct collecting urine produced in several nephrons and carrying it to a calix.

肾小球
肾单位的一部分。保障血液的过滤和尿液的产生。肾小球由一簇毛细血管组成，这些毛细血管包裹在一个囊腔之内。
glomerulus
Part of the nephron ensuring the filtering of blood and production of urine; the glomerulus is made up of a cluster of capillaries inserted into a capsule.

肾小管
肾单位的一部分，将尿液输送到集合管。
renal tubule
Part of the nephron carrying urine to a collectinag duct.

过滤 | Filtration

每个肾脏含有大约100万个肾单位。人体的全部血液每45分钟就会过滤一遍，但人每天排尿却只有0.5升到2升，这是因为大部分滤液又被重新吸收了。

Each kidney contains about one million nephrons. The entire volume of blood in the body is filtered every 45 minutes, but only 0.5 to 2 liters of urine are eliminated per day, since most of the filtrate is reabsorbed.

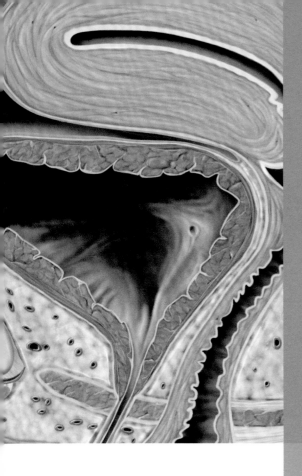

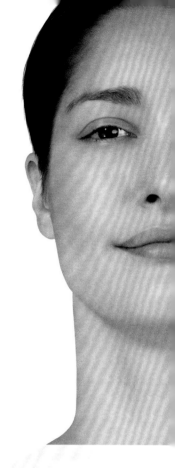

生殖系统 Reproductive system

生殖系统由多个生殖器官组成。男性和女性具有不同的生殖器官，包括生殖腺（睾丸、卵巢）、性腺（前列腺、精囊、前庭大腺）、生殖道（子宫、输卵管、阴道、输精管）和外部器官（阴茎、外阴）。生殖器官与生俱来，但只有到青春期，这些器官才会最终成形并发挥全部功能。乳房不是生殖器官，但在人类生殖中却非常重要（哺乳）。

The reproductive system is the group of organs that fulfill the reproduction function. These organs—the genital organs—are different in each sex and include the gonads (testicles, ovaries), the sexual glands (prostate, seminal vesicles, Bartholini glands), the genital tracts (uterus, uterine tubes, vagina, deferent ducts) and the external organs (penis, vulva). The genital organs are present at birth, but they become fully functional only at puberty, when they reach their final form. Breasts are not genital organs but play an important role in reproduction (breast feeding).

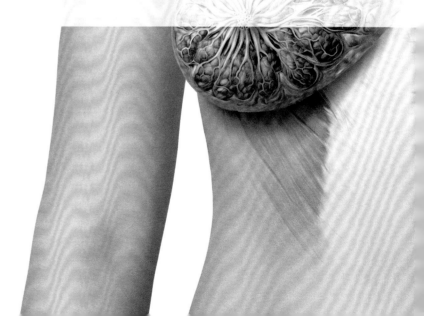

男性生殖器官

男性特有的器官，行使生殖功能。

male genital organs
Organs specific to men that ensure reproduction.

男性生殖器官矢状面
sagittal section of male genital organs

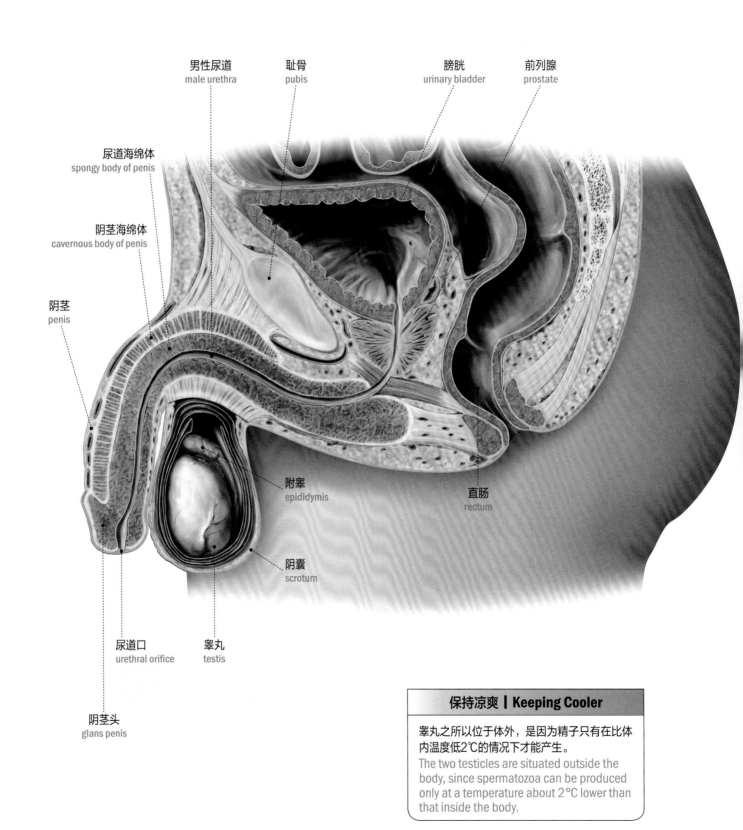

男性尿道
male urethra

耻骨
pubis

膀胱
urinary bladder

前列腺
prostate

尿道海绵体
spongy body of penis

阴茎海绵体
cavernous body of penis

阴茎
penis

附睾
epididymis

直肠
rectum

阴囊
scrotum

尿道口
urethral orifice

睾丸
testis

阴茎头
glans penis

保持凉爽 | Keeping Cooler

睾丸之所以位于体外，是因为精子只有在比体内温度低2℃的情况下才能产生。

The two testicles are situated outside the body, since spermatozoa can be produced only at a temperature about 2℃ lower than that inside the body.

男性尿道
起始于膀胱底，穿过前列腺，沿阴茎走行，止于尿道口。可排尿和射精。

male urethra
Channel originating at the base of the bladder, crossing the prostate and running along the penis to the urethral orifice; it allows urination and ejaculation.

尿道海绵体
可勃起的圆柱体组织。沿阴茎全长包绕着尿道。

spongy body of penis
Cylinder of erectile tissue surrounding the urethra along the length of the penis.

阴茎海绵体
可勃起的圆柱形器官。共有两根。构成阴茎的背部。

cavernous body of penis
Each of two cylindrical erectile organs forming the body of the posterior part of the penis.

阴茎
可勃起的男性器官。可性交和排尿。

penis
Erectile organ of men allowing copulation and voiding of urine.

阴茎头
球根状的锥形结构。位于阴茎末端，有包皮覆盖。

glans penis
Bulbous, cone-shaped structure at the end of the penis, covered with a foreskin.

尿道口
尿道的末端。可排尿和射精。

urethral orifice
Terminal part of the urethra allowing the evacuation of urine and ejaculation of sperm.

耻骨
髂骨的前部，在耻骨联合水平形成关节。

pubis
Front part of the iliac bone, articulated at the level of the pubic symphysis.

膀胱
中空器官。暂时收集肾脏产生的尿液，在排尿时通过尿道排空。

urinary bladder
Hollow organ in which urine produced in the kidneys temporarily collects; it empties through the urethra during urination.

前列腺
男性腺体。位于膀胱下方，其分泌物主要用以组成精液。

prostate
Male gland located beneath the bladder; its secretions are involved especially in the formation of sperm.

直肠
大肠的末端。与肛门外部相连，可使粪便通过。

rectum
Terminal segment of the large intestine, connecting with the outside of the anus and allowing defecation.

附睾
长而折叠的管道。精子射出前在此处发育成熟。

epididymis
Long canal folded on itself, in which spermatozoa reach maturity before ejaculation.

阴囊
皮肤包膜。容纳睾丸。

scrotum
Cutaneous envelope containing the testes.

睾丸
男性性腺。共有两个, 位于阴囊中, 可产生精子和分泌雄性激素(睾酮)。

testis
Each of the two male sex glands in the scrotum producing spermatozoa and secreting male hormones (testosterone).

阴茎横截面
cross section of the penis

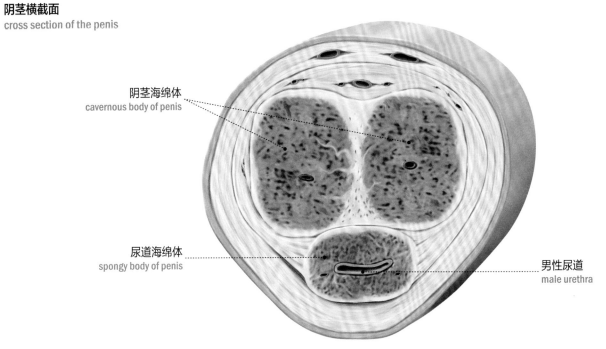

阴茎海绵体
cavernous body of penis

尿道海绵体
spongy body of penis

男性尿道
male urethra

睾丸剖面
section of the testis

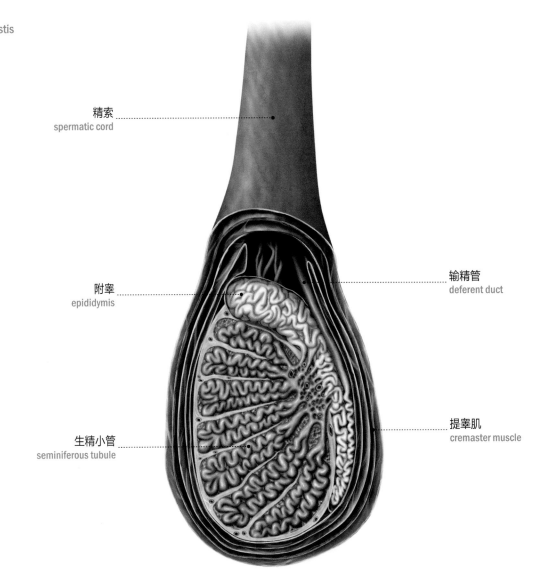

精索
spermatic cord

附睾
epididymis

输精管
deferent duct

提睾肌
cremaster muscle

生精小管
seminiferous tubule

阴茎海绵体
可勃起的圆柱形器官。共有两根，构成阴茎的背部。

cavernous body of penis
Each of two cylindrical erectile organs forming the body of the posterior part of the penis.

男性尿道
起始于膀胱底，穿过前列腺，沿阴茎走行，止于尿道口，可排尿和射精。

male urethra
Channel originating at the base of the bladder, crossing the prostate and running along the penis to the urethral orifice; it allows urination and ejaculation.

尿道海绵体
可勃起的圆柱体组织。沿阴茎全长包绕着尿道。

spongy body of penis
Cylinder of erectile tissue surrounding the urethra along the length of the penis.

精索
支撑睾丸和附睾的结构，其内有输精管、血管、淋巴管和神经。

spermatic cord
Structure supporting the testis and epididymis, containing the deferent duct and various blood and lymphatic vessels, as well as nerve threads.

输精管
将附睾中的精子输送到射精管的通道。

deferent duct
Canal carrying the spermatozoa of the epididymis to the ejaculatory duct.

附睾
长而折叠的管道。精子射出前在此处发育成熟。

epididymis
Long canal folded on itself, in which spermatozoa reach maturity before ejaculation.

提睾肌
包裹睾丸的肌肉，提睾肌收缩可使睾丸贴近身体，以提高温度。

cremaster muscle
Muscle enveloping the testes; its contraction allows them to be drawn near the body to warm them.

生精小管
位于睾丸中的小型管状结构，产生精子，然后将精子输送到附睾。

seminiferous tubule
Small tube located in the testes and producing the spermatozoa that are then carried to the epididymis.

女性生殖器官
女性特有的器官。行使生殖功能，分为外生殖器和内生殖器。

female genital organs
Organs specific to women that ensure reproduction; there are external organs and internal organs.

女性生殖器官前剖面
frontal section of female genital organs

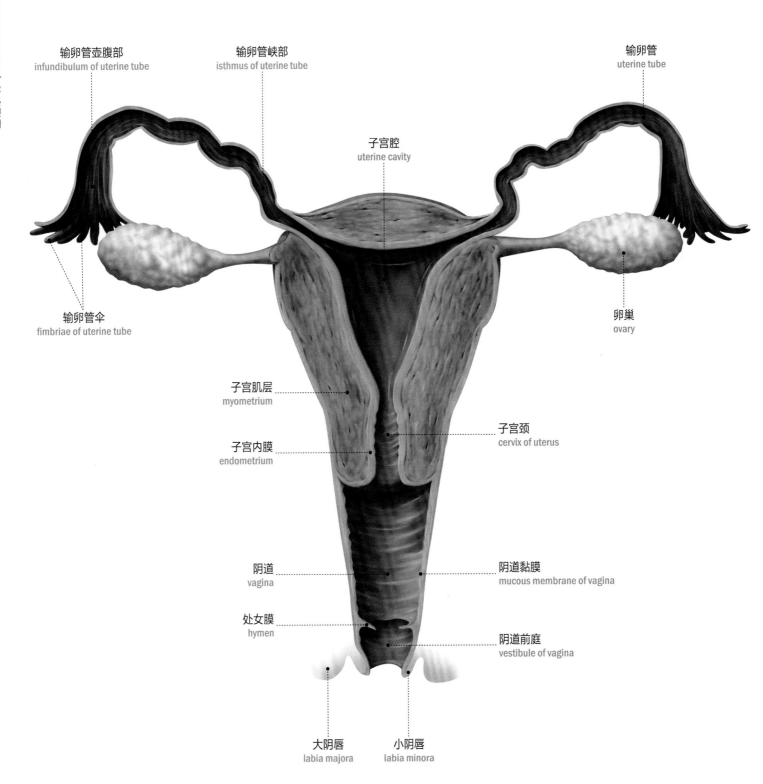

输卵管壶腹部
infundibulum of uterine tube

输卵管峡部
isthmus of uterine tube

输卵管
uterine tube

子宫腔
uterine cavity

输卵管伞
fimbriae of uterine tube

卵巢
ovary

子宫肌层
myometrium

子宫颈
cervix of uterus

子宫内膜
endometrium

阴道
vagina

阴道黏膜
mucous membrane of vagina

处女膜
hymen

阴道前庭
vestibule of vagina

大阴唇
labia majora

小阴唇
labia minora

输卵管峡部
输卵管的狭窄部分。开口于子宫。
isthmus of uterine tube
Narrow part of the uterine tube opening into the uterus.

子宫腔
由子宫壁围成空腔。
uterine cavity
Hollow space contained inside the walls of the uterus.

输卵管壶腹部
输卵管的漏斗状部分。卵子由此进入输卵管。
infundibulum of uterine tube
Funnel-shaped part of the uterine tube in which the ovum penetrates.

输卵管
开口于子宫上部（即子宫底）的两条管道。输卵管末端有伞状突起，能扫拂卵巢，拾集卵子。
uterine tube
Each of two tubes culminating in the upper part of the uterus and having fimbriae that sweep the ovaries and collect ova.

输卵管伞
输卵管的伞状延伸。在排卵时，输卵管伞毛能来回摆动并轻拂卵巢，产生涌流，从而将卵子推向输卵管。
fimbriae of uterine tube
Fringe-like extensions of the uterine tube, undulating and sweeping the ovary at the moment of ovulation to create a current that carries the ovum toward the tube.

卵巢
女性生殖腺体。分别位于子宫两侧，能产生卵细胞和性激素（雌激素和孕激素）。
ovary
Each of two female genital glands located on either side of the uterus, producing ova and sex hormones (estrogens and progesterone).

子宫肌层
子宫的肌壁。分娩时，子宫壁收缩以娩出婴儿。
myometrium
Muscular wall of the uterus contracting during childbirth to expel the baby.

子宫颈
子宫的下方末端。开口于阴道。
cervix of uterus
Lower extremity of the uterus opening into the vagina.

子宫内膜
被覆于子宫内部的黏膜。作用是接收受精卵，若无受精，部分内膜会破裂脱落，形成月经。
endometrium
Mucous membrane lining the inside of the uterus to receive the fertilized ovum; its partial destruction in the absence of fertilization causes menstruation.

阴道黏膜
充满褶皱的黏膜。被覆于阴道内壁，在性交时分泌滑液。
mucous membrane of vagina
Highly folded mucous membrane lining the wall of the vagina and secreting a lubricating substance during intercourse.

阴道
肌性管道。从子宫颈延伸到外阴，以便性交。
vagina
Muscular channel extending from the neck of the uterus to the vulva, allowing copulation.

阴道前庭
小阴唇间的间隙，阴道和尿道开口于此。
vestibule of vagina
Space between the labia minora through which the vagina and urethra open.

处女膜
细孔膜。由阴道黏膜的褶皱形成，将阴道与外阴隔开。
hymen
Fine perforated membrane formed by a fold of the vaginal mucous membrane, separating the vagina from the vulva.

大阴唇
皮肤褶皱。包围外阴，保护阴道口。
labia majora
Cutaneous folds bounding the vulva and protecting the vaginal opening.

小阴唇
皮肤褶皱。位于大阴唇内侧。
labia minora
Cutaneous folds located inside the labia majora.

卵巢周期

一系列事件过程。涉及卵母细胞的成熟和释放，也涉及其周围的卵泡组织。卵巢周期由三个连续的阶段组成：卵泡期、排卵期和黄体期。

ovarian cycle
Series of events involving the maturation and liberation of the oocyte as well as the follicular tissue surrounding it. It consists of three successive phases: the follicular phase, the ovulatory phase and the luteal phase.

卵泡期
follicular phase

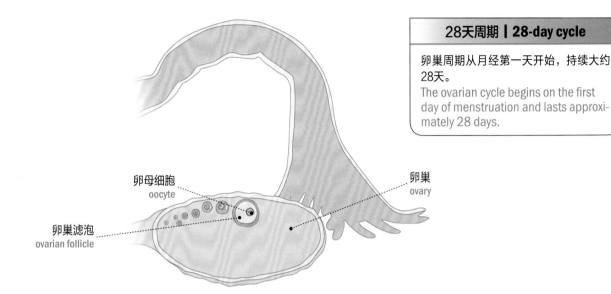

28天周期 ❘ 28-day cycle
卵巢周期从月经第一天开始，持续大约28天。 The ovarian cycle begins on the first day of menstruation and lasts approximately 28 days.

卵母细胞
oocyte

卵巢
ovary

卵巢滤泡
ovarian follicle

排卵期
ovulatory phase

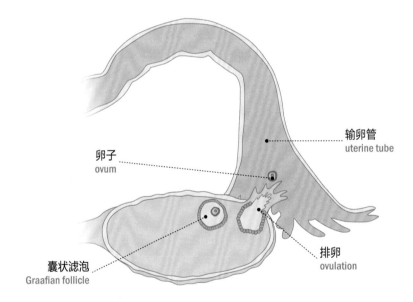

输卵管
uterine tube

卵子
ovum

囊状滤泡
Graafian follicle

排卵
ovulation

黄体期
luteal phase

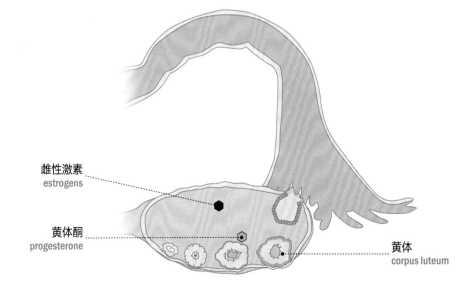

雌性激素
estrogens

黄体酮
progesterone

黄体
corpus luteum

卵母细胞

女性生殖细胞。处于生长发育阶段，下一阶段成为成熟卵子。

oocyte

Female sex cell in growth stage that is evolving toward a fertile ovule state.

卵巢滤泡

卵巢里的腔体。供卵母细胞在内发育。

ovarian follicle

Cavity of the ovary in which an oocyte develops.

卵子

成熟的女性生殖细胞。由卵巢产生，受精后，可使胚胎发育。

ovum

Mature female reproductive cell produced by the ovary; after fertilization by a spermatozoon, it enables an embryo to develop.

囊状滤泡

卵泡。含有成熟的卵母细胞，等待排往输卵管。排卵后被称为卵子。

Graafian follicle

Ovarian follicle containing a mature oocyte ready to be expelled into the fallopian tube. After ovulation, it is called an ovule.

雌性激素

性激素。由卵巢分泌，调节生殖器官的发育、月经后子宫内膜的再生。

estrogens

Sex hormones secreted by the ovaries, which govern the development of the genital organs and the renewal of the endometrium after menstruation.

黄体酮

性激素。由黄体和胎盘分泌，主要功能是为妊娠做准备。

progesterone

Sex hormone secreted by the corpus luteum and the placenta and whose principal function is to prepare for gestation.

卵巢

女性生殖腺体。分别位于子宫两侧，能产生卵细胞和性激素（雌激素和孕激素）。

ovary

Each of two female genital glands located on either side of the uterus, producing ova and sex hormones (estrogens and progesterone).

输卵管

开口于子宫上部（即子宫底）的两条管道。输卵管末端有伞状突起，能扫拂卵巢，收集卵子。

uterine tube

Each of two tubes culminating in the upper part of the uterus and having fimbriae that sweep the ovaries and collect ova.

排卵

卵子被卵巢排出并被输卵管末端的输卵管伞拾取的现象。

ovulation

Phenomenon in which an ovule is expelled by the ovary and grasped by the fringed extremity of the Fallopian tube.

黄体

临时的内分泌腺。可分泌黄体酮，如卵子未受精，黄体会在卵巢周期结束时退化。黄体是从囊状卵泡在释放卵母细胞后发展而来的。

corpus luteum

Temporary endocrine gland that secrets progesterone and that degenerates at the end of the ovarian cycle if the ovule is not fertilized. It develops from a Graafian follicle liberated from its oocyte.

女性生殖器矢状面
sagittal section of female genital organs

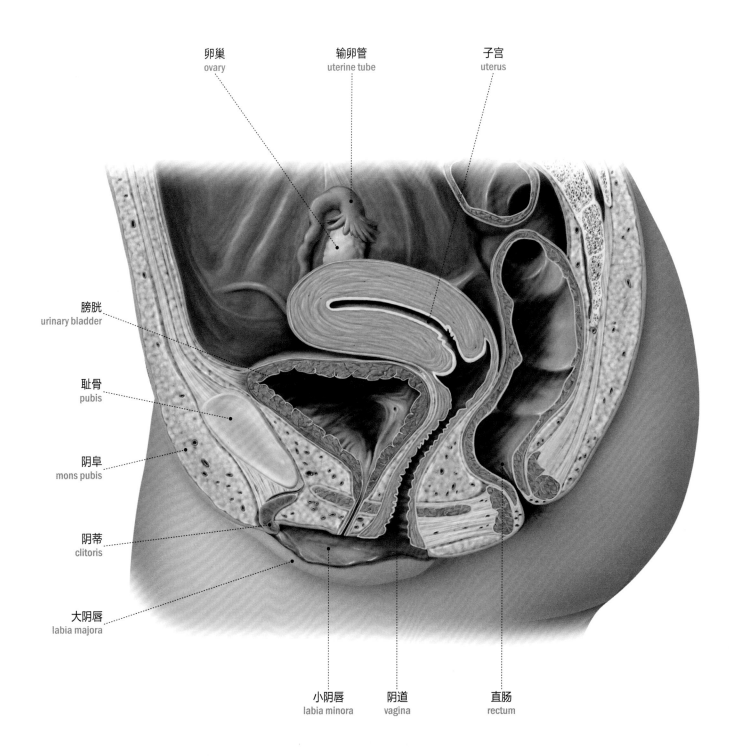

卵巢
ovary

输卵管
uterine tube

子宫
uterus

膀胱
urinary bladder

耻骨
pubis

阴阜
mons pubis

阴蒂
clitoris

大阴唇
labia majora

小阴唇
labia minora

阴道
vagina

直肠
rectum

卵巢

女性生殖腺体。分别位于子宫两侧，能产生卵细胞和性激素（雌激素和孕激素）。

ovary

Each of two female genital glands located on either side of the uterus, producing ova and sex hormones (estrogens and progesterone).

膀胱

中空器官。暂时收集肾脏产生的尿液，排尿时通过尿道排空。

urinary bladder

Hollow organ in which urine produced in the kidneys temporarily collects; it empties through the urethra during urination.

输卵管

开口于子宫上部（即子宫底）的两条管道。输卵管末端有伞状突起，能扫拂卵巢，收集卵子。

uterine tube

Each of two tubes culminating in the upper part of the uterus and having fimbriae that sweep the ovaries and collect ova.

耻骨

髂骨前部。在耻骨联合水平形成关节。

pubis

Front part of the iliac bone, articulated at the level of the pubic symphysis.

子宫

女性生殖器官，位于膀胱和直肠之间，怀孕期间胎儿在此发育。

uterus

Female genital organ located between the bladder and the rectum, in which the fetus develops during pregnancy.

阴阜

脂肪组织。覆盖耻骨，形成保护垫。

mons pubis

Adipose tissue covering the pubis and forming a protective cushion.

小阴唇

皮肤褶皱。位于大阴唇内侧。

labia minora

Cutaneous folds located inside the labia majora.

阴蒂

可勃起的小器官。有丰富的神经和静脉，形成重要的敏感区。

clitoris

Small erectile organ richly innervated and veined, forming an important erogenous zone.

阴道

肌性管道。从子宫颈延伸到外阴，以便性交。

vagina

Muscular channel extending from the neck of the uterus to the vulva, allowing copulation.

大阴唇

皮肤褶皱。包围外阴，保护阴道口。

labia majora

Cutaneous folds bounding the vulva and protecting the vaginal opening.

直肠

大肠的末端。与肛门外部相连，粪便通过直肠后排出。

rectum

Terminal segment of the large intestine, connecting with the outside of the anus and allowing defecation.

乳房

腺体器官。富含脂肪组织，包裹着胸肌，可分泌乳汁，哺乳新生儿。

breasts

Glandular organs rich in adipose tissue, enclosing the pectoral muscles and secreting milk to feed the newborn after birth.

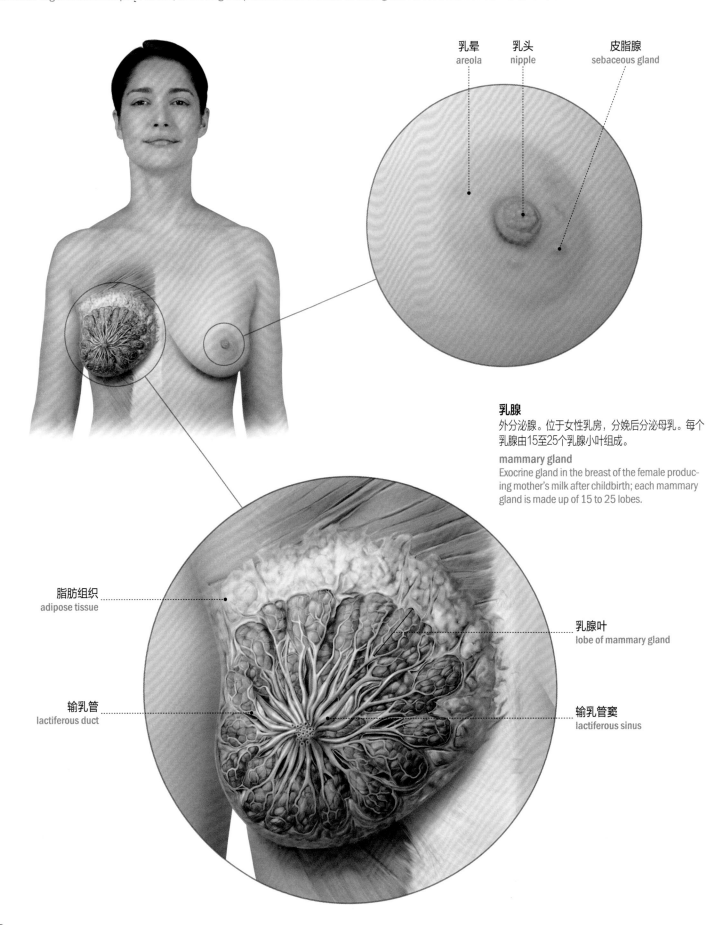

乳晕
areola

乳头
nipple

皮脂腺
sebaceous gland

乳腺

外分泌腺。位于女性乳房，分娩后分泌母乳。每个乳腺由15至25个乳腺小叶组成。

mammary gland

Exocrine gland in the breast of the female producing mother's milk after childbirth; each mammary gland is made up of 15 to 25 lobes.

脂肪组织
adipose tissue

乳腺叶
lobe of mammary gland

输乳管
lactiferous duct

输乳管窦
lactiferous sinus

多胞胎 | Doubling Up

多胎妊娠是指两个及以上胎儿在子宫内同时发育。多胎有两种类型，来自两种不同的过程：同卵双胎来自同一个卵子，而异卵双胎来自两个单独的受精卵。

A multiple pregnancy is the simultaneous development of more than one fetus in the uterus. There are two types of multiple pregnancies, resulting from very different processes. Identical twins come from a single ovum, while fraternal twins come from two separate fertilized_ova.

乳晕
围绕乳头的色素沉着区域。

areola
Pigmented area surrounding the nipple.

乳头
乳房的突出部分。可挺起，呈圆锥形或圆柱形，周围有乳晕。对女性来说，乳头也是输乳管的出口。

nipple
Erectile projection of the breast, cone-shaped or cylindrical, surrounded by the areola; in the female, the nipple is also the outlet of the lactiferous ducts.

皮脂腺
外分泌腺。多与毛囊相接，在皮肤表面排出皮脂。

sebaceous gland
Exocrine gland often associated with a hair follicle, excreting sebum at the surface of the skin.

脂肪组织
主要由脂肪细胞组成的结缔组织。是能量的储备地和体温的源泉。是人体正常运转不可或缺的物质。

adipose tissue
Connective tissue mainly formed of adipocytes; an energy reserve and source of warmth, it is indispensable for the functioning of the body.

乳腺叶
乳腺的一部分。在输乳管窦分泌乳汁。由许多小叶组成。

lobe of mammary gland
Part of the mammary gland secreting milk in the lactiferous sinuses; it is formed of numerous small lobules.

输乳管
将乳腺分泌的乳汁输送到乳头的通道。

lactiferous duct
Channel carrying milk secreted by the mammary gland to the nipple.

输乳管窦
输乳管的扩大部分。两次哺乳间期，乳汁积聚于此。

lactiferous sinus
Enlargement of the lactiferous duct in which mother's milk accumulates between two feedings.

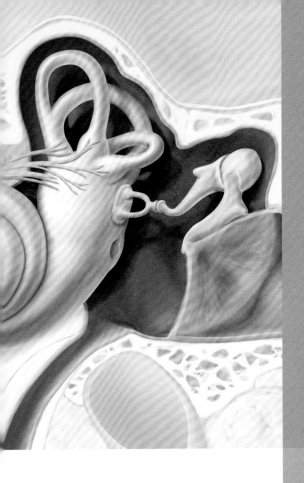

感觉器官 Sense organs

感觉是指人体通过神经系统感知和分析外部世界的多种功能。人类有五种感觉：视觉、听觉、嗅觉、味觉和触觉。感觉通过位于特定器官（眼睛，耳朵，鼻腔，舌，皮肤）上的感受器，来处理不同类型的物理刺激（光，声音，压力，温度、重力等）和化学刺激（嗅觉分子和味觉分子）。

The senses are body functions that enable the nervous system to perceive and analyze the outside world. Human beings have five senses: sight, hearing, smell, taste, touch. The senses process different types of physical (light, sound, pressure, temperature, gravity, etc.) and chemical (smell and taste molecules) stimuli through sensory receptors located in specific organs (eyes, ears, nasal cavity, tongue, skin).

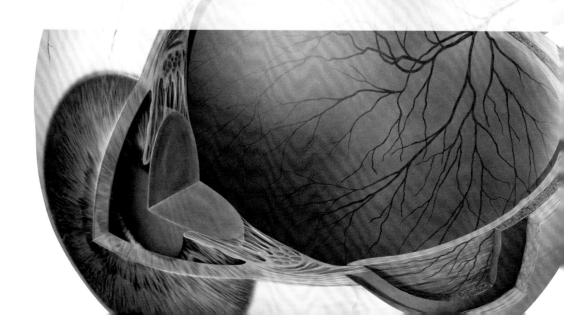

视觉 | sight

视觉

感觉的一种。光线刺激被眼睛感受，并被解析为对物体颜色、形状、距离和速度的有意识认知。

sight

Sense by which light stimuli perceived by the eyes are interpreted into conscious perceptions of an object's color, shape, distance and speed.

眼球

视觉器官。球形，位于眼眶内。捕捉光信号并传送到脑部，以供形成图像。

eyeball

Spherical-shaped organ of sight housed in the orbit; it captures light signals and transmits them to the brain to be formed into images.

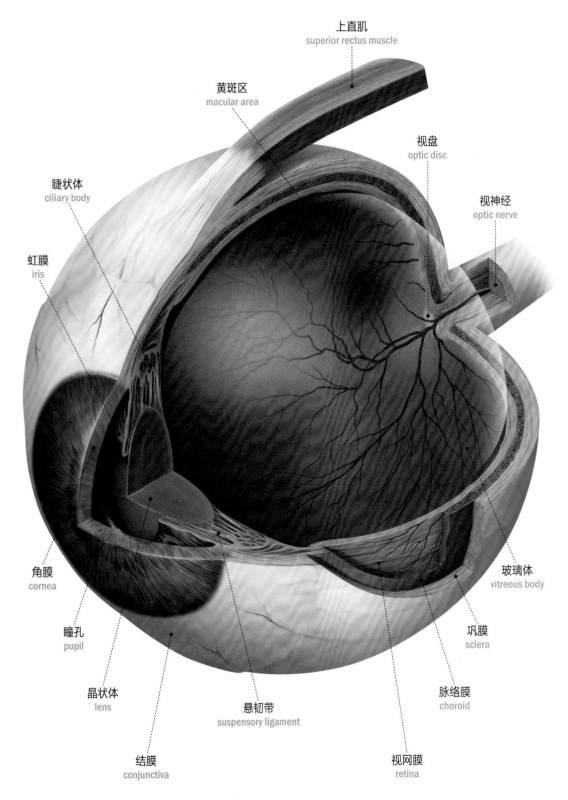

上直肌
superior rectus muscle

黄斑区
macular area

视盘
optic disc

视神经
optic nerve

睫状体
ciliary body

虹膜
iris

角膜
cornea

玻璃体
vitreous body

瞳孔
pupil

巩膜
sclera

晶状体
lens

悬韧带
suspensory ligament

脉络膜
choroid

结膜
conjunctiva

视网膜
retina

睫状体

肌肉组织。包绕在晶状体周围，通过改变自身形状，来调节晶状体的适应性。

ciliary body
Muscle tissue surrounding the lens and changing its shape to allow the lens to adapt.

虹膜

眼球表面的有色部分。由平滑肌组成，平滑肌可不自主收缩，因而改变瞳孔直径。

iris
Colored part of the surface of the eye, made up of smooth muscles whose involuntary contraction changes the diameter of the pupil.

角膜

透明的圆拱形膜。位于眼睛前部，可折射进入眼球的光线。

cornea
Transparent dome-shaped membrane located in the front of the eye, refracting light rays.

瞳孔

虹膜中心的圆孔。其孔径大小可变，以调节进入眼睛光线的多少。

pupil
Circular aperture at the centre of the iris; its opening varies to regulate the amount of light entering the eye.

晶状体

透明的柔韧纤维圆盘。位于虹膜后面，作为可变透镜，折射光线。

lens
Transparent flexible fibrous disk located behind the iris, acting as a variable lens refracting light rays.

结膜

透明黏膜。覆盖在眼睛的前表面，但不覆盖角膜，可产生润滑黏液。

conjunctiva
Transparent mucous membrane covering the front surface of the eye, except the cornea, and producing lubricating mucus.

悬韧带

连接睫状体和晶状体的韧带。使晶状体在眼球内固定。

suspensory ligament
Ligament connecting the ciliary body to the lens keeping it in place inside the eyeball.

黄斑区

位于视网膜中心的小型区域，靠近视盘。此处成像最清晰。

macular area
Small area located at the centre of the retina, near the optic disk, where visual acuity is best.

上直肌

可使眼球向上运动的肌肉。

superior rectus muscle
Muscle allowing the eyeball to move upward.

视盘

视网膜上没有光感受器的区域。血管和神经纤维在此聚集，形成视神经。

optic disc
Region of the retina with no photoreceptors, where blood vessels and nerve fibers gather to form the optic nerve.

视神经

感觉神经。负责视觉，将信息从眼睛传递到脑。

optic nerve
Sensory nerve responsible for vision: it transmits information from the eye to the encephalon.

玻璃体

透明胶状物。充满眼睛内部，以维持其球体形状。

vitreous body
Transparent gelatinous substance filling the eye and assisting in maintaining its spherical shape.

巩膜

不透明的白色纤维结缔组织，保护和支撑眼睛结构。

sclera
Opaque white fibrous connective tissue, protecting and supporting the structure of the eye.

脉络膜

富含血管的膜。覆盖视网膜。

choroid
Membrane rich in blood vessels covering the retina.

视网膜

眼球的内膜。由数以百万计的感光细胞组成，将光信号转换成神经信号。

retina
Inner membrane of the eye, made up of millions of photoreceptors that transform light into nerve signals.

眼

视觉器官。用于感知形状、距离、颜色和
运动。

eye
Organ of vision serving to perceive shapes,
distances, colors and movements.

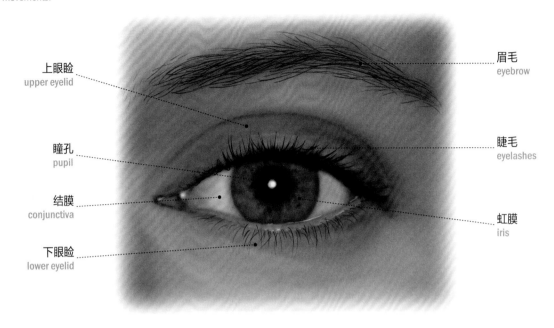

上眼睑
upper eyelid

眉毛
eyebrow

瞳孔
pupil

睫毛
eyelashes

结膜
conjunctiva

虹膜
iris

下眼睑
lower eyelid

视网膜

眼球的内膜。由数以百万计的感光细胞
组成，将光转换成神经信号。

retina
Inner membrane of the eye, made
up of millions of photoreceptors that
transform light into nerve signals.

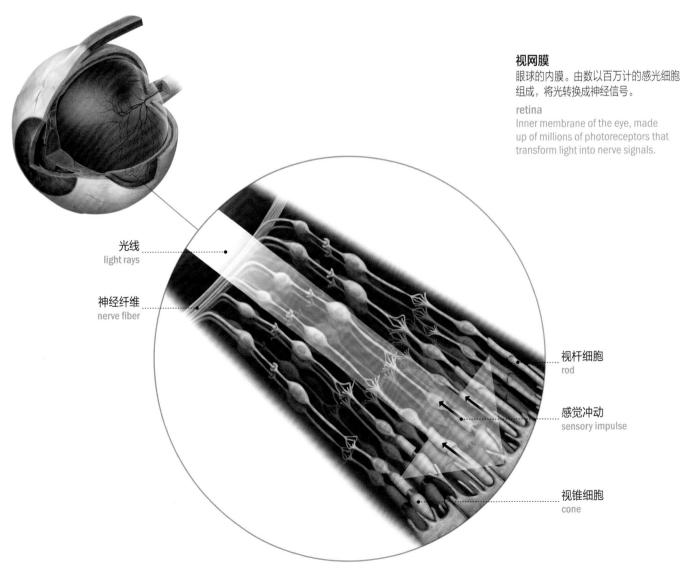

光线
light rays

神经纤维
nerve fiber

视杆细胞
rod

感觉冲动
sensory impulse

视锥细胞
cone

上眼睑
起于眼睛上缘的眼睑。上眼睑比下眼睑要大一些，活动也更灵活一些。

upper eyelid
Eyelid rising from the upper edge of the eye; it is larger and more mobile than the lower eyelid.

瞳孔
虹膜中心的圆孔。其孔径大小可变，以调节进入眼睛的光线多少。

pupil
Circular aperture at the centre of the iris; its opening varies to regulate the amount of light entering the eye.

结膜
透明黏膜。覆盖在眼睛的前表面，但不覆盖角膜，可产生润滑黏液。

conjunctiva
Transparent mucous membrane covering the front surface of the eye, except the cornea, and producing lubricating mucus.

下眼睑
起于眼睛下缘的眼睑。

lower eyelid
Eyelid rising from the lower edge of the eye.

眉毛
两眼上方的拱形毛发。

eyebrow
Arched area of hair above each eye.

睫毛
长于眼睑外缘的毛发。可防止灰尘和其他异物落入眼睛。

eyelashes
Hairs on the outer edge of the eyelids, preventing dust and other foreign particles from depositing on the eye.

虹膜
眼球表面的有色部分。由平滑肌组成，平滑肌可不自主收缩，因而改变瞳孔直径。

iris
Colored part of the surface of the eye, made up of smooth muscles whose involuntary contraction changes the diameter of the pupil.

眨眼 | Blink of an Eye

我们会经常眨眼，主要目的是使眼睛表面保持湿润。平均每天会眨5 400次，其中眼睑的总闭合时间约为30分钟。

The blinking of eyelids, the main purpose of which is to humidify the surface of the eye, occurs very frequently. On average, eyelids blink 5,400 times per day–a total of about 30 minutes with the eyelids closed.

光线
由物体发出或由其反射的光束，穿过视网膜，可刺激感光细胞（视锥细胞和视杆细胞）。

light rays
Rays emitted or reflected by an object, crossing the retina and stimulating the photoreceptors (cones and rods).

神经纤维
运动神经或感觉神经的轴突。在神经内以成束的形式存在。

nerve fiber
Axon of a motor or sensory nerve, grouped into a fascicle inside a nerve.

视杆细胞
感光细胞。负责外围和光强度较低时的视觉。对色彩不敏感。

rod
Photoreceptor responsible for peripheral and low-intensity light vision but not sensitive to colors.

感觉冲动
电信号。由视网膜上的感光细胞（光感受器）发出。

sensory impulse
Electrical signal produced by light-sensitive cells (photoreceptors) located on the retina.

视锥细胞
对色彩敏感的感光细胞。在光强度较高时，有助于提供图像细节。

cone
Color-sensitive photoreceptor assisting in supplying detailed images but requiring strong light intensity.

眼外肌

小肌肉。共有6块，通过肌肉收缩，可使眼睛在眼眶内运动。

extraocular muscles
Small muscles (6) whose contraction causes the eye to move in its orbit.

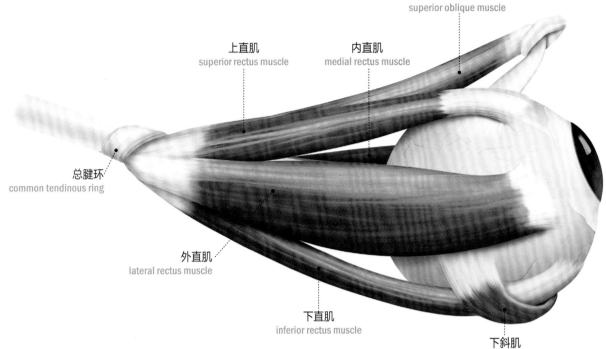

上斜肌
superior oblique muscle

上直肌
superior rectus muscle

内直肌
medial rectus muscle

总腱环
common tendinous ring

外直肌
lateral rectus muscle

下直肌
inferior rectus muscle

下斜肌
inferior oblique muscle

视觉原理

角膜和晶状体能够折射来自物体的光线，从而可在视网膜上投射出清晰的图像。感光细胞将这种光信号转换成神经信号，再通过视神经传输到大脑。

mechanism of vision
The cornea and lens refract light from an object in order to project a clear image on the retina; photoreceptors transform this light signal into a nerve signal that is transmitted to the brain through the optic nerve.

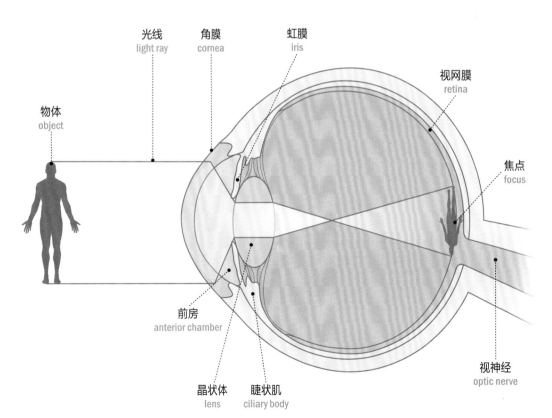

光线
light ray

角膜
cornea

虹膜
iris

视网膜
retina

物体
object

焦点
focus

前房
anterior chamber

晶状体
lens

睫状肌
ciliary body

视神经
optic nerve

上直肌
连接总腱环到巩膜上部的肌肉。可使眼球向上运动。

superior rectus muscle
Muscle connecting the common tendinous ring to the upper part of the sclera; it allows upward movement of the eyeball.

内直肌
连接总腱环到巩膜内侧的肌肉。可使眼球向内运动。

medial rectus muscle
Muscle connecting the common tendinous ring to the inner part of the sclera; it allows adduction of the eyeball.

上斜肌
连接蝶骨和巩膜的肌肉。可使眼球下旋和内旋。

superior oblique muscle
Muscle connecting the sphenoid bone to the sclera; it allows downward and inward rotation of the eyeball.

总腱环
环形肌腱。眼外肌的共用止点，位于眼眶后部，与蝶骨相连。

common tendinous ring
Common insertion tendon of the rectus muscles of the eye at the back of the orbit, attached to the sphenoid bone.

外直肌
连接总腱环到巩膜外侧的肌肉。可使眼球向外运动。

lateral rectus muscle
Muscle connecting the common tendinous ring to the outer part of the sclera; it allows outward movement of the eyeball.

下直肌
连接总腱环到巩膜下部的肌肉。可使眼球向下运动。

inferior rectus muscle
Muscle connecting the common tendinous ring to the lower part of the sclera; it allows downward movement of the eyeball.

下斜肌
连接上颌骨和巩膜的肌肉。可使眼球上旋和外旋。

inferior oblique muscle
Muscle connecting the maxilla to the sclera; it allows upward and outward rotation of the eyeball.

物体
物体发出的光线。穿过眼睛的不同区域后，在视网膜上形成颠倒的图像。

object
Light rays emitted by an object cross the different areas of the eye to form a reverse image on the retina.

角膜
透明的圆拱形膜。位于眼睛前部，可使进入眼球的光线发生折射。

cornea
Transparent dome-shaped membrane located in the front of the eye, refracting light rays.

视网膜
眼睛的内膜。由数以百万计的光感受器组成，将光转换成神经信号。

retina
Inner membrane of the eye, made up of millions of photoreceptors that transform light into nerve signals.

视神经
感觉神经。负责把视觉信息从眼睛传递到脑。

optic nerve
Sensory nerve responsible for vision: it transmits information from the eye to the encephalon.

晶状体
透明的柔韧纤维圆盘。位于虹膜后面，作为可变透镜，折射光线。

lens
Transparent flexible fibrous disk located behind the iris, acting as a variable lens refracting light rays.

光线
物体发出的光所走过的路线。

light ray
Line along which light emitted by an object flows through.

虹膜
眼睛表面的有色部分。由平滑肌组成，平滑肌可不自主收缩，因而改变瞳孔直径。

iris
Colored part of the surface of the eye, made up of smooth muscles whose involuntary contraction changes the diameter of the pupil.

焦点
光线在该点汇聚，形成图像，在正常视力下，焦点位于视网膜上。

focus
Point where light rays converge and the image is formed; in normal vision, the focus is on the retina.

睫状体
包绕在晶状体周围的肌肉组织。通过改变自身形状，来调节晶状体的适应性。

ciliary body
Muscle tissue surrounding the lens and changing its shape to allow the lens to adapt.

前房
角膜和虹膜之间的空隙，充满滋养性液体——房水。

anterior chamber
Space between the cornea and iris filled with a nourishing fluid, aqueous humor.

视觉缺陷

图像未能形成在视网膜上，导致视力模糊。可通过戴眼镜、隐形眼镜或手术加以矫正。

vision defects

The image does not form on the retina, resulting in blurred vision that is corrected by wearing glasses or contact lenses, or by surgery.

近视
myopia

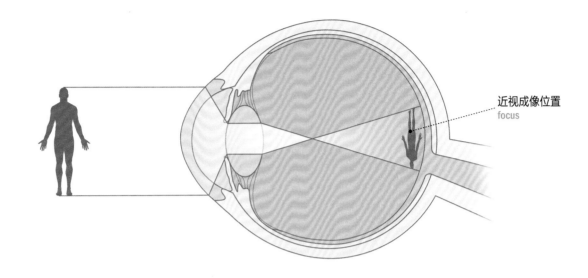

近视成像位置
focus

远视
hyperopia

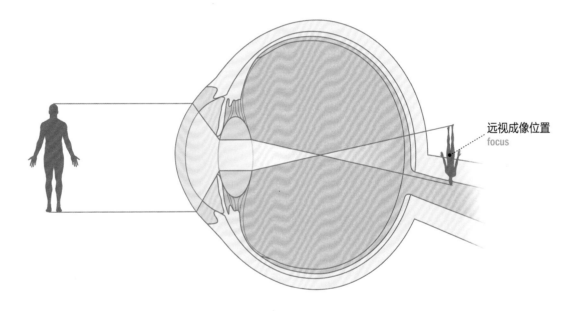

远视成像位置
focus

散光
astigmatism

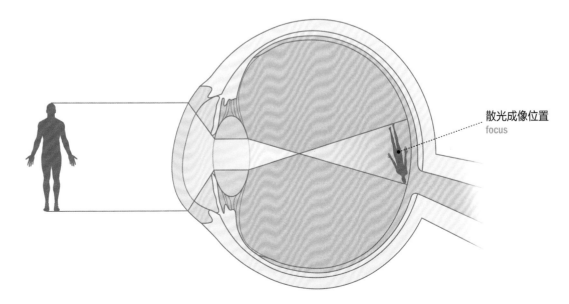

散光成像位置
focus

近视

视力缺陷。特征是难以清楚辨别远处的物体，这是由于晶状体不能正常聚焦光线而引起的。

myopia
Vision defect characterized by difficulty distinguishing faraway objects; it is caused by the faulty convergence of light rays by the lens.

近视成像位置

光线在焦点汇聚而成图像，在近视的情况下，焦点位于视网膜之前。

focus
Point where light rays converge and the image is formed; in the case of myopia, the image forms in front of the retina.

远视

视力缺陷。特征是难以清楚辨别近处的物体，这是由于晶状体不能正常聚焦光线而引起的。

hyperopia
Vision defect characterized by difficulty distinguishing close objects clearly; it is caused by the faulty convergence of light rays by the lens.

远视成像位置

光线在焦点汇聚而成图像，在远视的情况下，焦点位于视网膜之后。

focus
Point where light rays converge and the image is formed; in the case of hypermetropia, the image forms behind the retina.

散光

视力缺陷。特征是在不同的轴线上，无论远近都视力模糊，这通常是由角膜的屈光缺陷造成的。

astigmatism
Vision defect characterized by blurred vision, near or far, based on different axes; it is generally caused by the faulty curvature of the cornea.

散光成像位置

由于眼球在各个不同子午线上的屈光力不同，平行光经眼屈光系统后不能形成焦点。

focus
The light is bent in more than one direction, so objects appear blurry and not fully in focus.

立体图像 | Three Dimensions

由于两只眼睛观察物体的角度略有不同，这使得我们大脑能够估算物体的距离和景深，从而形成立体视觉。

Each of the two eyes perceives objects from a slightly different angle. This enables the brain to assess distance and depth, thus providing three-dimensional vision.

听觉

感觉的一种。耳朵感受到声音的振动，大脑将其解析为声音。

hearing

Sense by which sound vibrations are perceived by the ear and interpreted as sounds by the brain.

耳

既是听觉器官，也是平衡器官。分为三部分：外耳、中耳和内耳。

ear

Organ of hearing and balance made up of three parts: the outer ear, the middle ear and the inner ear.

外耳外侧观

external ear: lateral view

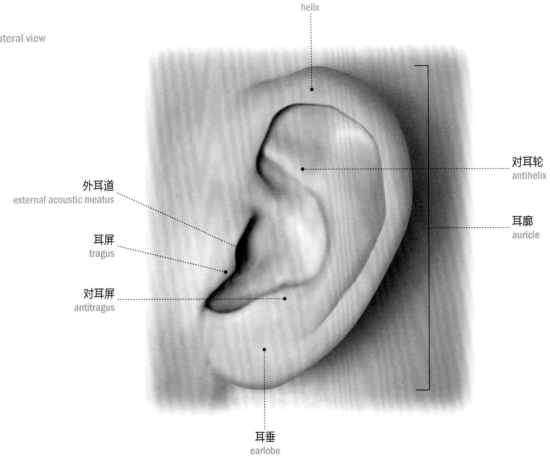

耳轮
helix

对耳轮
antihelix

耳廓
auricle

外耳道
external acoustic meatus

耳屏
tragus

对耳屏
antitragus

耳垂
earlobe

外耳

耳朵的一部分。可收集声音振动并传导至中耳。

external ear

Part of the ear collecting sound vibrations and directing them to the middle ear.

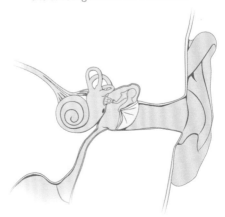

中耳

充满空气的空腔。可将外耳捕捉到的声音振动传递到内耳。

middle ear

Air-filled cavity transmitting sound vibrations captured by the external ear to the internal ear.

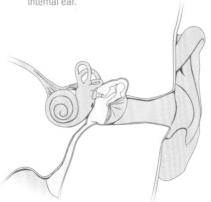

内耳

腔体。由多个液囊和导管组成，包含听觉器官和平衡器官。

internal ear

Cavity formed of a series of fluid-filled sacs and ducts; it contains the sensory organs of hearing and balance.

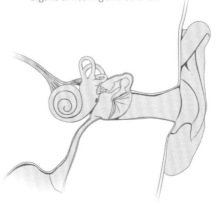

倾听万籁 | Thousands of Sounds

耳朵能分辨出近四十万种不同的声音。声音的强度以分贝为单位来计量。耳朵的可听阈值设为0分贝，而疼痛阈值为120分贝（相当于飞机起飞时的声音）。

The ears distinguish almost 400,000 different sounds, the intensity of which is measured in decibels. The audibility threshold is set at 0 dB, while the pain threshold corresponds to 120 dB (the sound of an airplane taking off).

外耳道
骨性通道。耳廓捕捉到的声音由此到达鼓膜。

external acoustic meatus
Bony canal through which sounds captured by the pinna reach the eardrum.

耳屏
扁平的三角形突起。位于外耳道开口的前面。

tragus
Flat triangular eminence in front of the opening of the external auditory meatus.

对耳屏
小的三角形突起。位于对耳轮的下末端。

antitragus
Small triangular eminence at the lower extremity of the antihelix.

耳垂
外耳丰满的末端，没有软骨。

earlobe
Fleshy extremity of the external ear, having no cartilage.

耳轮
耳廓的边缘。

helix
Rim of the auricle of the ear.

对耳轮
耳廓上的突起。平行于耳轮，上部分分成两支。

antihelix
Prominence of the auricle of the ear, parallel to the helix; its upper part is divided into two branches.

耳廓
纤维软骨体。锥形，可捕捉声音振动并将其引导至外耳道。

auricle
Fibrocartilaginous cone capturing sound vibrations and directing them to the external auditory meatus.

耳的剖面图
section of ear

前庭
vestibule

半规管
semicircular canals

前庭神经
vestibular nerve

耳蜗神经
cochlear nerve

颞骨
temporal bone

外耳道
external acoustic meatus

砧骨
incus

镫骨
stapes

锤骨
malleus

耳蜗
cochlea

鼓膜
tympanic membrane

咽鼓管
auditory tube

听力机制
耳廓捕捉声音振动并将其引导至外耳道，在那里引起鼓膜振动。三块听骨将振动放大后传递到耳蜗，耳蜗再将振动转换为神经冲动。

mechanism of hearing
The auricle captures sound vibrations and directs them to the external auditory meatus where they make the tympanic membrane vibrate; the three ossicles amplify them and transmit them to the cochlea that then transforms them into a nerve impulse.

耳蜗神经
cochlear nerve

卵圆窗
oval window

听小骨
ossicles

声振动
sound vibrations

外耳道
external acoustic meatus

外淋巴液
perilymph

神经纤维
nerve fiber

螺旋器
organ of Corti

耳蜗导管
cochlear duct

耳蜗
cochlea

蜗窗
round window

鼓膜
tympanic membrane

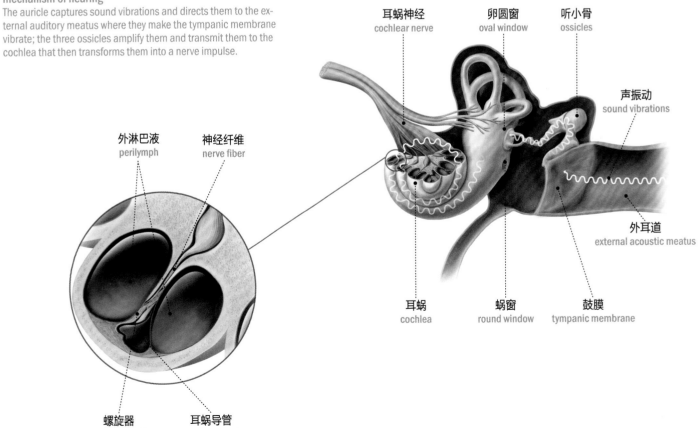

前庭神经

前庭耳蜗神经的分支。负责身体平衡。

vestibular nerve
Branch of the vestibulocochlear nerve responsible for balance.

耳蜗神经

前庭耳蜗神经的分支。负责听觉。

cochlear nerve
Branch of the vestibulocochlear nerve responsible for hearing.

颞骨

成对的骨。位于颅骨外侧，与下颌骨的分支相连。

temporal bone
Paired bone in the lateral part of the skull articulating with the branches of the mandible.

耳蜗

听觉的感觉器官。由一个螺旋管组成，里面充满着液体，可接收听骨的振动并转换为神经冲动。

cochlea
Sensory organ of hearing, formed of a spiral tube filled with fluids; it receives the vibrations of the ossicles and transforms them into nerve impulses.

前庭

内耳的骨性空腔。负责静态平衡（当人站立不动时）。

vestibule
Bony cavity of the internal ear responsible for static balance (when standing immobile).

半规管

内耳的骨性管道。负责控制身体平衡，共有三条，每一条都与空间的一个维度相对应。

semicircular canals
Bony canals in the internal ear responsible for controlling balance; each of the three canals is associated with a dimension of space.

鼓膜

结缔组织薄膜。封闭中耳入口处，可将声音振动传递给听骨。

tympanic membrane
Thin membrane of connective tissue closing the entrance to the middle ear and transmitting the sound vibrations to the ossicles.

咽鼓管

狭窄管道。连接中耳和咽部，调节鼓膜两侧的压力。

auditory tube
Narrow tube connecting the middle ear to the pharynx and regulating the pressure on either side of the tympanic membrane.

外耳道

骨性通道。耳廓捕获的声音由此到达鼓膜。

external acoustic meatus
Bony canal through which sounds captured by the pinna reach the eardrum.

砧骨

与锤骨和镫骨相连的听小骨。

incus
Ossicle articulating with the malleus and stapes.

锤骨

与鼓膜接触的听小骨。

malleus
Ossicle in contact with the tympanic membrane.

镫骨

可把砧骨的振动传递给耳蜗的听小骨。

stapes
Ossicle transmitting the vibrations of the incus to the cochlea.

外淋巴液

含于内耳的骨性腔室的液体。

perilymph
Fluid contained in the bony compartments of the internal ear.

神经纤维

运动神经或感觉神经的轴突。在神经内以成束的形式存在。

nerve fiber
Axon of a motor or sensory nerve, grouped into a fascicle inside a nerve.

螺旋器

由感觉细胞形成的器官。它能检测到外淋巴液的运动并将其转化为神经信号。

organ of Corti
Organ formed of sensory cells that detect the movements of the perilymph and transform them into nerve signals.

耳蜗导管

耳蜗的中央管道，由膜包围而成。内部充满内淋巴液。

cochlear duct
Central canal of the cochlea bounded by membranes and filled with a fluid called endolymph.

耳蜗神经

前庭耳蜗神经的分支。负责听觉。

cochlear nerve
Branch of the vestibulocochlear nerve responsible for hearing.

卵圆窗

耳蜗出口。镫骨坐落于此，声音的振动可以穿透它。

oval window
Outlet of the cochlea against which the stapes rests; sound vibrations penetrate through it.

听小骨

位于中耳腔内的小骨头，共有三块。负责放大声音振动。

ossicles
Small bones (3) housed in the cavity of the middle ear and responsible for amplifying sound vibrations.

声振动

sound vibrations

外耳道

骨性通道。耳廓捕获的声音由此到达鼓膜。

external acoustic meatus
Bony canal through which sounds captured by the pinna reach the eardrum.

鼓膜

结缔组织薄膜。封闭中耳入口处，可把声音振动传递给听骨。

tympanic membrane
Thin membrane of connective tissue closing the entrance to the middle ear and transmitting the sound vibrations to the ossicles.

蜗窗

耳蜗出口。在刺激螺旋器后，声音振动由此离开耳蜗。

round window
Outlet through which sound vibrations leave the cochlea after stimulating the organ of Corti.

耳蜗

听觉的感觉器官。由一个螺旋管组成，里面充满着液体，可接收听骨的振动并转换为神经冲动。

cochlea
Sensory organ of hearing, formed of a spiral tube filled with fluids; it receives the vibrations of the ossicles and transforms them into nerve impulses.

嗅觉

感觉的一种。负责感知气味。

smell

Sense by which odors are perceived.

鼻腔矢状面

鼻腔：鼻腔由鼻中隔一分为二，前方开口于鼻孔，后方开门于咽部。

sagittal section of nasal cavity

Nasal cavities: each of two cavities, separated by the nasal septum and opening in front through the nostrils and in back into the pharynx.

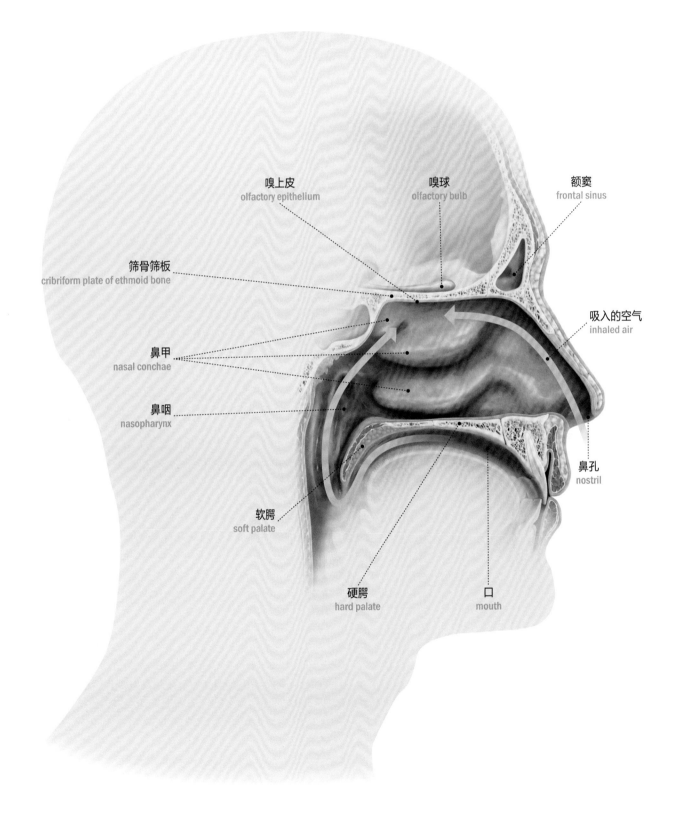

嗅上皮
olfactory epithelium

嗅球
olfactory bulb

额窦
frontal sinus

筛骨筛板
cribriform plate of ethmoid bone

吸入的空气
inhaled air

鼻甲
nasal conchae

鼻咽
nasopharynx

鼻孔
nostril

软腭
soft palate

硬腭
hard palate

口
mouth

再生 | Regeneration

嗅细胞似乎是人体中唯一一种能够再生的神经元。其生存周期约为60天。

Olfactory cells are apparently the only neurons in the human body capable of regeneration. They have a life span of about 60 days.

嗅上皮

嗅觉感受器。位于鼻腔顶部，由数以百万计的嗅觉细胞组成。受到气味分子的刺激可产生神经信号。

olfactory epithelium
Sensory organ of smell lining the roof of the nasal cavities; it consists of millions of olfactory cells whose stimulation by odorous molecules generates a nerve signal.

筛骨筛板

筛骨的下部。嗅神经由此通过。

cribriform plate of ethmoid bone
Lower side of the ethmoid bone through which the olfactory nerves pass.

鼻甲

鼻腔外侧壁的骨性延伸。对吸入的空气加热加湿。

nasal conchae
Bony extensions of the lateral wall of the nasal cavities, serving to warm and humidify inhaled air.

鼻咽

咽的上部。与鼻腔相连。

nasopharynx
Upper part of the pharynx connecting with the nasal cavities.

软腭

肌膜壁。分隔咽部与口腔，主要作用是帮助摄取食物和发声。

soft palate
Muscular membranous wall separating the pharynx and buccal cavity; it assists especially in ingestion of food and vocalization.

嗅球

神经组织的膨大部分。连接着嗅神经，起中继作用，负责把嗅觉信息传递给大脑。

olfactory bulb
Enlargement of nerve tissue connected to the olfactory nerves; it serves as a relay in transmitting olfactory information to the cerebrum.

额窦

额骨上的空腔。与鼻腔相连，加热吸入的空气。

frontal sinus
Cavity in the frontal bone, connecting with the nasal cavities and warming inhaled air.

吸入的空气

inhaled air

鼻孔

开口。空气由此进入鼻腔。

nostril
Orifice of the nose through which air enters the nasal cavities.

口

消化道的起始段。由嘴唇包围着的口腔组成，可消化食物，并在味觉、说话和呼吸中发挥作用。

mouth
Initial part of the digestive tube made up of a cavity (oral cavity) surrounded by lips; it allows the ingestion of food and plays a role in tasting, speaking and breathing.

硬腭

骨性分隔。口腔与鼻腔的分界，由软腭延伸而来。

hard palate
Bony separation between the buccal and nasal cavities, extended by the soft palate.

嗅觉机制

气味分子进入鼻腔，溶解在鼻黏液中，刺激嗅细胞。嗅细胞产生神经信号，由嗅神经传递给大脑。

mechanism of smell
Odorous molecules entering the nasal cavities are dissolved in the nasal mucus, then stimulating the olfactory cells that generate nerve signals transmitted to the brain by the olfactory nerves.

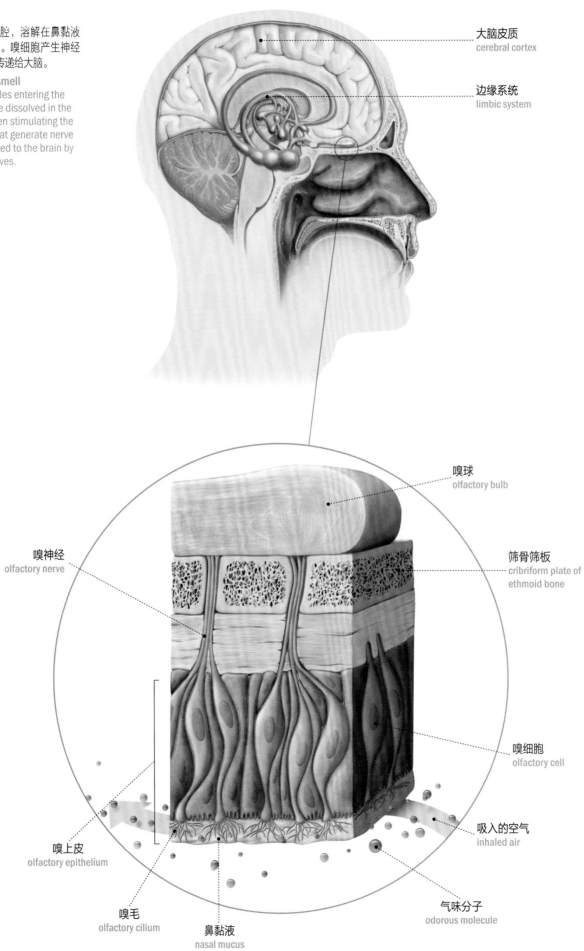

大脑皮质
cerebral cortex

边缘系统
limbic system

嗅球
olfactory bulb

嗅神经
olfactory nerve

筛骨筛板
cribriform plate of ethmoid bone

嗅细胞
olfactory cell

吸入的空气
inhaled air

气味分子
odorous molecule

嗅上皮
olfactory epithelium

嗅毛
olfactory cilium

鼻黏液
nasal mucus

大脑皮质
大脑半球的表层。可感知并有意识地分析气味。

cerebral cortex
Superficial layer of the cerebral hemispheres, in which smells are perceived and consciously analyzed.

边缘系统
所有的可将感知到的气味与情感和记忆联系起来的神经结构。

limbic system
All the nerve structures associating perceived smells with emotions and memories.

嗅神经
感觉神经。负责嗅觉。

olfactory nerve
Sensory nerve involved in smell.

嗅球
神经组织的膨大部分。连接着嗅神经，起中继作用，负责把嗅觉信息传递给大脑。

olfactory bulb
Enlargement of nerve tissue connected to the olfactory nerves; it serves as a relay in transmitting olfactory information to the cerebrum.

嗅上皮
位于鼻腔顶部的嗅觉感受器。由数以百万计的嗅觉细胞组成，受到气味分子的刺激可产生神经信号。

olfactory epithelium
Sensory organ of smell lining the roof of the nasal cavities; it consists of millions of olfactory cells whose stimulation by odorous molecules generates a nerve signal.

筛骨筛板
筛骨的下部。嗅神经由此通过。

cribriform plate of ethmoid bone
Lower side of the ethmoid bone through which the olfactory nerves pass.

嗅毛
嗅觉细胞树突的微细末端。内含感受器。

olfactory cilium
Fine extension of the dendrite of an olfactory cell containing a receptor.

嗅细胞
感觉神经元。构成嗅觉感受器，它们的轴突聚集在一起，组成嗅神经。

olfactory cell
Each of the sensory neurons constituting olfactory receptors; their axons come together to form olfactory nerves.

鼻黏液
黏稠半透明物质。由鼻腔黏膜产生。

nasal mucus
Viscous translucent substance produced by the mucous membrane of nasal cavities.

吸入的空气
inhaled air

气味分子
挥发性化学物质。在空气中传播并可产生气味。

odorous molecule
Volatile chemical substance transported in the air and causing odors.

味觉 | taste

味觉

感觉的一种。可感知进入嘴内东西的味道，其主要功能是提供关于食物特性的信息，触发消化液的分泌。

taste

Sense by which the flavor of substances placed in the mouth is perceived; its main functions are to provide information about food quality and to trigger the secretion of digestive juices.

舌上面观
舌：口腔的肌性器官。负责味觉、咀嚼和说话。

tongue: superior view
Tongue: muscular organ in the buccal cavity involved in tasting, chewing and speaking.

颚扁桃体
淋巴器官。共有两个，位于口腔后部。有抑菌功能，可保护呼吸道。

palatine tonsil
Each of two lymphoid organs located behind the buccal cavity, protecting the airways by fighting bacteria.

舌扁桃体
淋巴器官。共两个，位于舌根底部。具有免疫功能。

lingual tonsil
Each of the two lymphoid organs located at the base of the tongue, contributing to the immune defense.

界沟
V形槽。将舌的活动部分与固定部分隔开。

terminal sulcus
A V-shaped groove separating the mobile part from the fixed part of the tongue.

舌正中沟
沿着舌头全长的一道凹陷。将舌头分为对称的两半。

median lingual sulcus
Depression extending the full length of the tongue and dividing it into two symmetrical halves.

菌状乳头
味觉乳头。红色圆形，位于舌头表面。主要感知甜味和咸味。

fungiform papilla
Round red gustatory papilla on the surface of the tongue; it reacts mostly to sweet and salty tastes.

会厌
软骨瓣。位于喉的上部，可活动，在吞咽时刻引导食物进入食管。

epiglottis
Mobile catilaginous lamina located in the upper part of the larynx, directing food to the esophagus at the moment of swallowing.

盲孔
小凹陷。位于界沟的顶部。

foramen cecum
Small depression located at the summit of the terminal sulcus.

轮廓乳头
大型味觉乳头。位于舌头后部，主要感知苦味。

circumvallate papilla
Large gustatory papilla located behind the tongue; it perceives mostly bitter tastes.

叶状乳头
味觉乳头。条纹状，位于舌两侧。对酸味尤其敏感。

foliate papilla
Striated gustatory papilla located on the sides of the tongue; it is mostly sensitive to acidic tastes.

舌黏膜
覆盖舌的黏膜。主要由丝状乳头构成，使其具有天鹅绒般柔软的外观。

mucous membrane of tongue
Mucous membrane covering the tongue and made up mainly of filiform papillae that give it a velvety appearance.

舌尖
舌的末端。可灵活移动。

apex of tongue
Mobile extremity of the tongue.

轮廓乳头
大型味觉乳头。位于舌后部，它主要感知苦味。

circumvallate papilla
Large gustatory papilla located behind the tongue; it perceives mostly bitter tastes.

丝状乳头
锥形乳头。位于舌背，功能仅限于触觉。

filiform papilla
Cone-shaped papilla located on the back of the tongue; its function is solely tactile.

舌表面截面
舌的表面散布着小突起，称为乳头。乳头内含味蕾。

section of tongue's surface
Surface of the tongue dotted with small protuberances called papillae, containing taste buds.

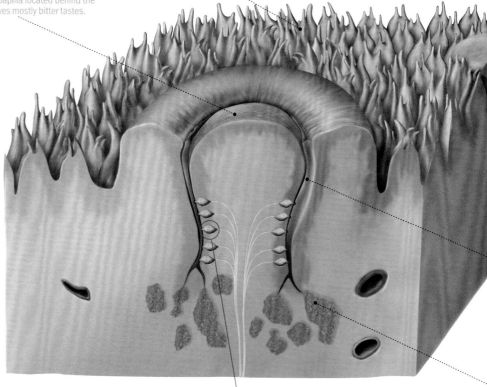

唾液
略显黏稠的液体。由口腔内的唾液腺分泌，主要含消化酶。

saliva
More or less viscous fluid secreted in the mouth by the salivary glands; it contains especially a digestive enzyme.

唾液腺
外分泌腺。可分泌唾液，大量存在于舌的黏膜之中。

salivary gland
Exocrine gland secreting saliva, present in large numbers in the mucous membrane of the tongue.

上皮
由紧密排列的上皮细胞形成的组织。

epithelium
Tissue formed of tightly packed epithelial cells.

味蕾
由大约100个味觉细胞形成的小器官，聚集在味觉乳头的上皮组织中。

taste bud
Small organ formed from some 100 taste cells, clustered in the epithelial tissue of a gustatory papilla.

味觉细胞
味蕾中的细胞。接触到有味物质时可产生神经信号。

taste cell
Cell located in a taste bud and generating a nerve signal when it comes into contact with a taste substance.

神经纤维
运动神经或感觉神经的轴突。在神经内以成束的形式存在。

nerve fiber
Axon of a motor or sensory nerve, grouped into a fascicle inside a nerve.

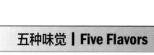

五种味觉 | Five Flavors

味觉感受器只能分辨出五种基本味道：甜、咸、酸、苦和鲜。鲜味是因为谷氨酸钠，例如酱油就有鲜味。

Taste receptors distinguish only five basic flavors: sweet, salty, acid, bitter, and umami. The last, associated with monosodium glutamate, is found, for instance, in soy sauce.

触觉 | touch

触觉

感觉的一种。通过与皮肤和某些黏膜的直接接触，能感知物体和环境的某些物理特性，如压力、温度和质地。

touch

Sense by which certain physical properties of objects and the environment (pressure, temperature, texture) are perceived through direct contact with the skin and certain mucous membranes.

皮肤

弹性防护器官。覆盖整个身体，主要分三层：表皮层、真皮层和皮下组织层。

skin

Flexible resistant organ covering the entire body, consisting of three main layers: the epidermis, dermis and hypodermis.

皮肤截面

皮肤含有大量触觉感受器。感受器分为若干种类。通常一种感受器专门感知一种特定刺激。

section of skin

Skin contains many tactile receptors. There are several types, generally specialized in perceiving a particular stimulus.

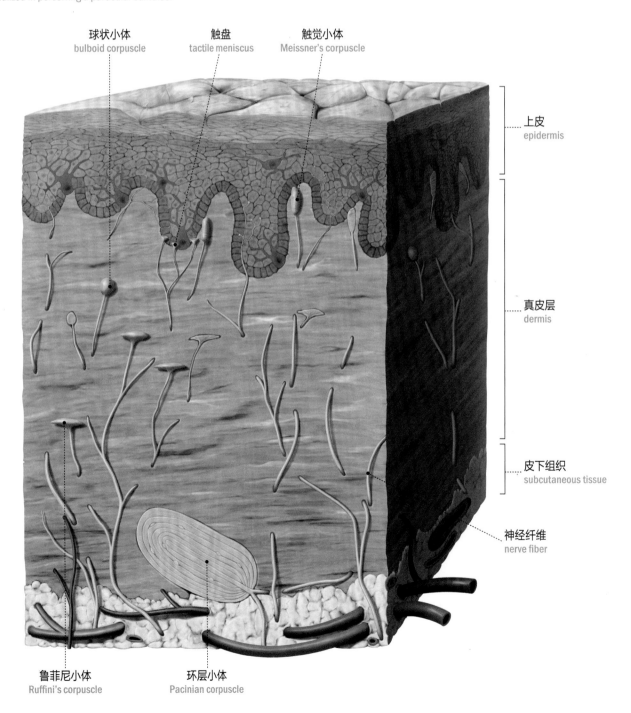

球状小体
bulboid corpuscle

触盘
tactile meniscus

触觉小体
Meissner's corpuscle

上皮
epidermis

真皮层
dermis

皮下组织
subcutaneous tissue

神经纤维
nerve fiber

鲁菲尼小体
Ruffini's corpuscle

环层小体
Pacinian corpuscle

球状小体
触觉感受器。位于真皮层，可感知特定触碰和寒冷。
bulboid corpuscle
Tactile receptor located in the dermis, sensitive to specific touch and cold.

上皮
皮肤的最外层。由上皮组织组成。
epidermis
Epithelial tissue forming the outermost part of the skin.

触盘
触觉感受器。位于表皮深层，可感知轻微触碰和刺痛。
tactile meniscus
Tactile receptor located in the deep layer of the epidermis, sensitive to light touch and acute pain.

真皮层
皮肤的中间层。位于表皮层之下，由富含胶原纤维和弹性纤维的结缔组织组成。
dermis
Middle layer of the skin, beneath the epidermis, formed of connective tissue rich in collagen fibers and elastic fibers.

触觉小体
触觉感受器。位于皮肤敏感部位（手、脚、嘴唇、生殖器）的真皮上部。可感知特定触碰。
Meissner's corpuscle
Tactile receptor located in the upper part of the dermis of sensitive areas (hands, feet, lips and genital organs), stimulated by specific touch.

皮下组织
皮肤的最内层。位于真皮层之下，富含脂肪。
subcutaneous tissue
Deep layer of the skin, beneath the dermis and rich in fat.

鲁菲尼小体
触觉感受器。位于有毛区域的真皮层和关节囊，可感知持续高压和暖热。
Ruffini's corpuscle
Tactile receptor located in the dermis of hairy regions and articular capsules, sensitive to strong continuous pressure and heat.

神经纤维
运动神经或感觉神经的轴突。在神经内以成束的形式存在。
nerve fiber
Axon of a motor or sensory nerve, grouped into a fascicle inside a nerve.

环层小体
触觉感受器。位于真皮深处，可感知持续强烈振动和压力。
Pacinian corpuscle
Tactile receptor located in the deep dermis, sensitive to strong continuous vibrations and pressure.

上皮截面
section of epidermis

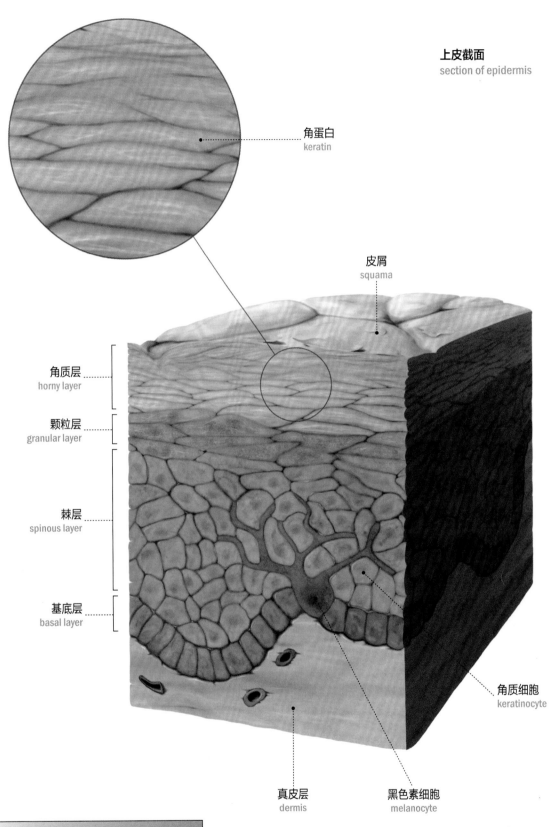

角蛋白
keratin

皮屑
squama

角质层
horny layer

颗粒层
granular layer

棘层
spinous layer

基底层
basal layer

角质细胞
keratinocyte

真皮层
dermis

黑色素细胞
melanocyte

死细胞 | Dead Cells

每年都有3~4千克的老化皮肤从身体表面脱落。也就是说，人体表皮每35到45天就会全部更换一次。

Each year, from 3 to 4 kg of worn skin detaches from the surface of the body. Thus, the epidermis is completely replaced every 35 to 45 day.

角蛋白

纤维蛋白。尤见于表皮、指甲和毛发的角质层，可限制皮肤脱水，形成屏障，抵御外部感染源。

keratin
Fibrous protein, especially abundant in the horny layer of the epidermis, nails and hairs, limiting dehydration of the skin and forming a barrier against external infectious agents.

角质层

表皮的浅表层。由失去细胞核的死亡角质细胞组成。

horny layer
Superficial layer of the epidermis formed of dead keratinocytes that have lost their nucleus.

皮屑

表皮的碎片。由死细胞组成，即将从角质层脱落。

squama
Small fragment of the epidermis made up of dead cells, detaching from the horny layer.

颗粒层

表皮的一层。由没有细胞活性的角质细胞组成，在到达角质层之前，角质细胞会变得扁平并使角蛋白聚集。

granular layer
Layer of epidermis consisting of keratinocytes with no cell activity that flatten and concentrate keratin before reaching the horny layer.

角质细胞

表皮的主要细胞。基底层不断产生角质细胞，然后迁移到棘层，在棘层生产和储存角蛋白。

keratinocyte
Main cell of the epidermis; constantly produced in the basal layer, it then migrates to the spinous layer where it produces and stockpiles keratin.

棘层

表皮的一层。主要由角质细胞组成，角质细胞逐渐富含角质和黑色素。

spinous layer
Layer of the epidermis consisting mainly of keratinocytes that progressively enrich themselves in keratin and melanin.

黑色素细胞

表皮的细胞。产生黑色素，这种色素决定了皮肤、眼睛的虹膜以及毛发的颜色。还可吸收紫外线，保护皮肤。

melanocyte
Cell of the epidermis that produces melanin, the pigment responsible for the color of the skin, iris of the eye and hair, playing a protective role against ultraviolet rays.

基底层

表皮的深层。位于与真皮的接触点，确保角质细胞的更新。

basal layer
Deep layer of the epidermis located at the contact point with the dermis, ensuring renewal of keratinocytes.

真皮层

皮肤的中间层。在表皮层之下，由富含胶原纤维和弹性纤维的结缔组织组成。

dermis
Middle layer of the skin, beneath the epidermis, formed of connective tissue rich in collagen fibers and elastic fibers.

毛发纵切面
毛发：富含角质的结构。附着在皮肤上，呈细丝状，柔软且有弹性。

longitudinal section of a hair
Hair: keratin-rich structure appended to the skin, having the shape of a very fine, flexible and resilient filament.

表皮层
毛发的外层。由富含角蛋白的细胞组成。像屋顶上的瓦片一样重叠在一起。

cuticle
Outer layer of the hair, made up of keratin-rich cells that overlap like shingles on a roof.

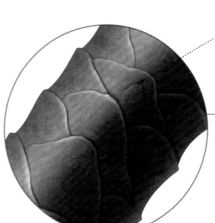

毛干
毛发在皮肤外的部分。形状纤细。

hair shaft
External part of hair at the slender end.

上皮
形成皮肤的最外层的上皮组织。

epidermis
Epithelial tissue forming the outermost part of the skin.

皮脂
黄色脂肪物质。由皮脂腺产生，可润滑和保护皮肤。

sebum
Fatty yellowish substance produced by the sebaceous glands, lubricating the skin and protecting it.

皮脂腺
外分泌腺。通常与毛囊相连，在皮肤表面分泌皮脂。

sebaceous gland
Exocrine gland often associated with a hair follicle, excreting sebum at the surface of the skin.

毛根
毛发在皮肤内的部分。

hair root
Part of the hair contained in the skin.

真皮层
皮肤的中间层。在表皮层之下，由富含胶原纤维和弹性纤维的结缔组织组成。

dermis
Middle layer of the skin, beneath the epidermis, formed of connective tissue rich in collagen fibers and elastic fibers.

毛球
毛囊的膨大末端。毛发在其内生长。

hair bulb
Enlarged end of the follicle from which the hair develops.

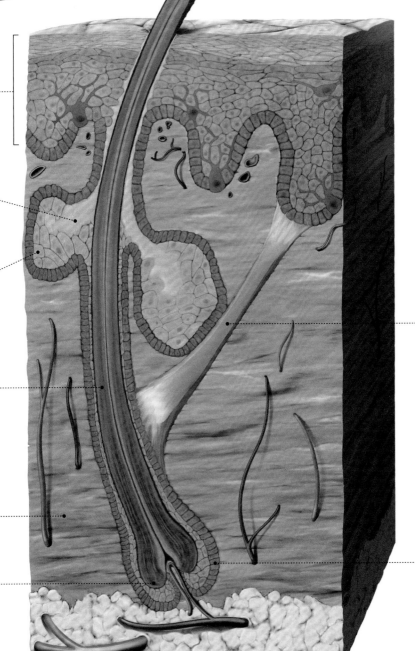

竖毛肌
绷紧的小肌肉。连接毛囊与表皮。可非自主收缩，使毛发直立。

arrector pili muscle
Tiny taut muscle between a hair follicle and the epidermis; its involuntary contraction causes the hair to stand up.

毛囊
真皮层内的包囊。毛发在其内生长。

hair follicle
Envelope inside the dermis, within which the hair develops.

手指截面

手指：手部的伸展部分。由若干关节连接的骨（指骨）构成，末端有指甲覆盖。

section of a finger
Finger: extension of the hand formed of various articulated bones (phalanges); its extremity is covered by a nail.

指甲

不停生长着的坚硬角质片。覆盖并保护手指和脚趾的远节指骨背侧。

nail
Continually-growing, hard horny plate covering and protecting the dorsum of the distal phalanges of the fingers and toes.

甲基质

表皮的一部分。指甲在其内生长。

nail matrix
Part of the epidermis from which the nail grows.

甲根

指甲的根部。甲根固定在甲基质中，由皮肤皱褶保护。

nail root
Base of the nail, anchored into the matrix and protected by a fold of skin.

甲弧影

指甲基底部的白色区域。在拇指上尤其明显。

lunula
White area at the base of the nail, especially visible on the thumb.

甲游离缘

带点白色的指甲末端。超过指尖。

free margin
Whitish extremity of the nail that extends beyond the tip of the finger.

甲床

指甲所依附的手指部分。含有丰富的血管，供应手指营养。

nail bed
Part of the finger on which the nail lies, containing numerous blood vessels that assure its nutrition.

真皮层

皮肤的中间层。在表皮层之下，由富含胶原纤维和弹性纤维的结缔组织组成。

dermis
Middle layer of the skin, beneath the epidermis, formed of connective tissue rich in collagen fibers and elastic fibers.

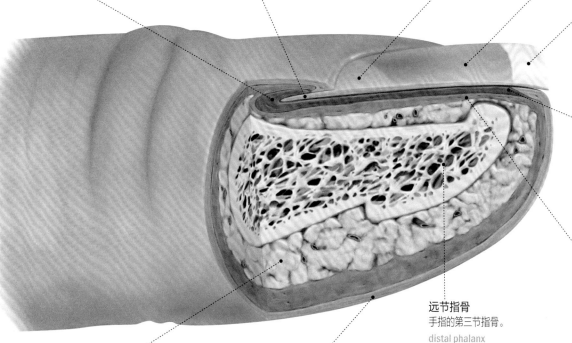

远节指骨

手指的第三节指骨。

distal phalanx
Third phalanx of the finger.

皮下组织

皮肤的深层。位于真皮层之下，富含脂肪。

subcutaneous tissue
Deep layer of the skin, beneath the dermis and rich in fat.

上皮

组成皮肤的最外层的上皮组织。

epidermis
Epithelial tissue forming the outermost part of the skin.

最大的器官 | The Biggest Organ

皮肤是人体最大和最重的器官，总面积约有2平方米，重5千克。其厚度在1.5~4毫米之间，不同部位厚度不一。

With a total area of about 2 square meters and a weight of 5 kg, the skin is the body's largest and heaviest organ. It is between 1.5 and 4 mm thick, depending on the area of the body.

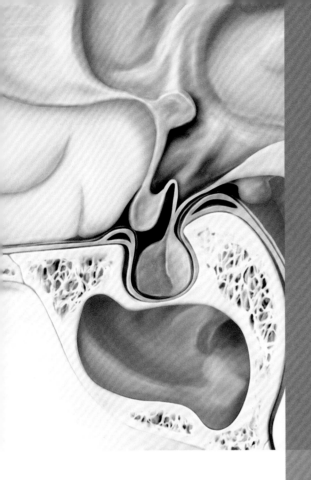

内分泌系统 Endocrine system

内分泌系统由多个腺体和细胞组成，通过释放一些化学物质进入血液，来调节身体的若干功能。这些化学物质称为激素。与中枢神经系统相配合，内分泌系统形成了人体的调节和反馈机制，来协调细胞的各种活动。内分泌系统在维持内环境稳定、新陈代谢、生长、生殖和应激反应等方面起着重要作用。

The endocrine system is a group of glands and cells that regulate certain body functions through chemical substances released into the blood: hormones. The endocrine system, in association with the central nervous system, forms a control and communication system that coordinates the cells' various activities. It plays a prominent role in maintaining homeostasis, metabolism, growth, reproduction, and response to stress.

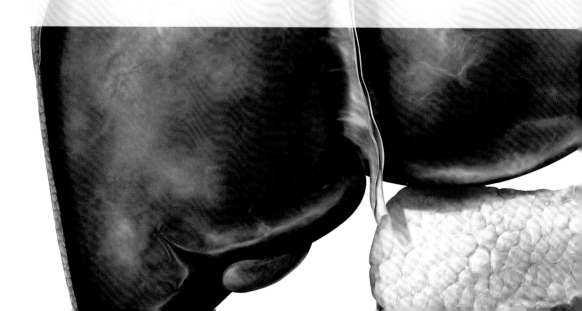

内分泌腺

腺体。可分泌激素进入血液，以特定方式作用于各种器官。

endocrine glands

Glands that secrete hormones, which are substances released into the bloodstream that act in specific ways on various organs.

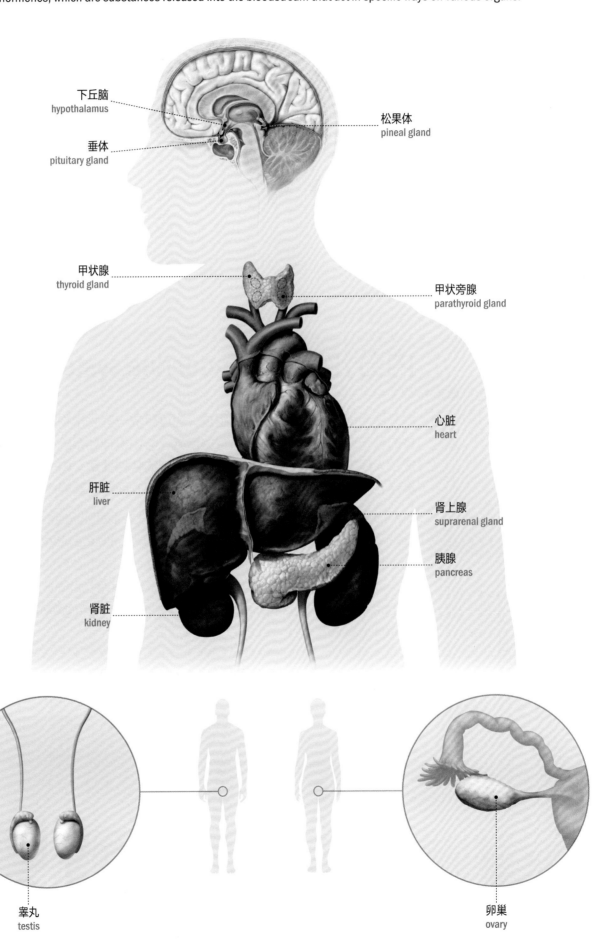

下丘脑
hypothalamus

松果体
pineal gland

垂体
pituitary gland

甲状腺
thyroid gland

甲状旁腺
parathyroid gland

心脏
heart

肝脏
liver

肾上腺
suprarenal gland

胰腺
pancreas

肾脏
kidney

睾丸
testis

卵巢
ovary

下丘脑
由灰质组成的小腺体。可调节垂体的激素分泌，控制自主神经系统活动。
hypothalamus
All the small formations of gray matter, controlling the hormonal secretions of the pituitary gland and the activity of the autonomic nervous system.

松果体
大脑的内分泌腺。可分泌褪黑素，影响精子形成或月经周期。
pineal gland
Endocrine gland of the brain secreting melatonin and influencing the formation of spermatozoa or the menstrual cycle.

垂体
内分泌腺。受下丘脑调控，可分泌9种主要激素。这些激素尤其针对生长、泌乳、血压和体液–水电解质平衡等发挥作用。
pituitary gland
Endocrine gland that is controlled by the hypothalamus and that secretes nine major hormones that act especially on growth, lactation, blood pressure and urine retention.

甲状旁腺
内分泌腺。位于甲状腺的后方，分泌的激素（甲状旁腺激素）可影响钙的代谢。
parathyroid gland
Each of the endocrine glands located behind the thyroid gland, secreting a hormone (parathyroid hormone) that acts on the calcium metabolism.

甲状腺
内分泌腺。位于喉和气管之间，可分泌与生长和代谢相关的激素（甲状腺激素和降钙素）。
thyroid gland
Endocrine gland that is located between the larynx and the trachea and that secretes hormones that act on growth and metabolism (thyroid hormones and calcitonin).

心脏
肌性器官。保障全身血液循环，可分泌一种激素，能抑制肾素分泌并调节醛固酮的活性。
heart
Muscular organ assuring blood circulation throughout the body; it secretes a hormone that inhibits renin secretion and modifies the action of aldosterone.

肝脏
大型腺体。在消化和代谢中起重要作用，肝脏尤可分泌与生长有关的一种激素（生长激素）。
liver
Large gland playing an important role in digestion and metabolism; the liver secretes especially a hormone (somatomedine) that is involved in growth.

肾上腺
内分泌腺。位于肾脏上方，可分泌多种激素，其中有的参与应激反应，有的参与体液平衡。
suprarenal gland
Endocrine gland located above the kidney; certain hormones that it secretes assist in the stress mechanism, while others act on water retention.

肾脏
位于腹腔内的一对器官。主要功能是产生尿液，也分泌肾素调节血压。
kidney
Each of two organs in the abdomen whose main function is to produce urine; it also secretes renin that regulates blood pressure.

胰腺
狭长型腺体。在消化食物（通过分泌胰液）和调节血糖（通过分泌胰岛素）中起着重要作用。
pancreas
Elongated gland playing an important role in digestion (secretion of pancreatic juices) and in control of blood sugar (secretion of insulin).

睾丸
2个男性性腺。位于阴囊中，可产生精子和分泌雄激素（睾酮）。
testis
Each of the two male sex glands in the scrotum producing spermatozoa and secreting male hormones (testosterone).

卵巢
一对女性生殖腺。位于子宫两侧，可产生卵细胞和性激素（雌激素和孕酮）。
ovary
Each of two female genital glands located on either side of the uterus, producing ova and sex hormones (estrogens and progesterone).

甲状腺

内分泌腺。位于喉和气管之间，可分泌与生长和代谢有关的激素（甲状腺激素和降钙素）。

thyroid gland
Endocrine gland that is located between the larynx and the trachea and that secretes hormones that act on growth and metabolism (thyroid hormones and calcitonin).

甲状腺前面观
thyroid gland: anterior view

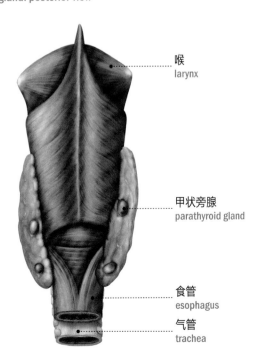

喉
larynx

甲状腺叶
lobe of the thyroid gland

甲状腺峡
isthmus of the thyroid gland

气管
trachea

甲状腺滤泡

甲状腺滤泡：小型球状结构。甲状腺的主要组成部分。

section of a thyroid follicle
Thyroid follicle: small spherical structure forming the major part of the thyroid gland.

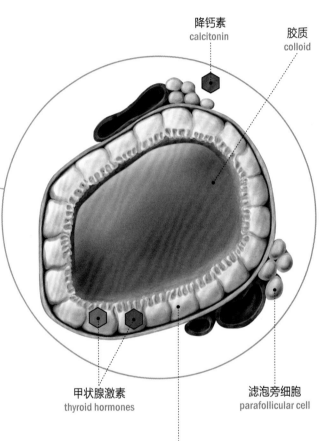

降钙素
calcitonin

胶质
colloid

甲状腺激素
thyroid hormones

滤泡细胞
follicular cell

滤泡旁细胞
parafollicular cell

甲状腺后面观
thyroid gland: posterior view

喉
larynx

甲状旁腺
parathyroid gland

食管
esophagus

气管
trachea

作用多种多样 | Various Roles

迄今为止，已分类的激素超过了一百种。激素的作用广泛而多样：可调节生长、生殖、身体对各种刺激（压力）的反应和新陈代谢等。

To date, more than a hundred hormones have been classified. Their effects are extensive and varied: they regulate growth, reproduction, the body's response to various stimuli (stress), metabolism, etc.

喉
肌性软骨通道。连接咽和气管，包含声带，具有发声和呼吸功能。

larynx
Muscular cartilaginous channel connecting the pharynx and trachea; it contains the vocal cords and has a vocalizing and respiratory function.

甲状腺叶
甲状腺的主要部分。共两叶，分别位于喉的两侧。

lobe of the thyroid gland
Each of two main parts of the thyroid gland, located on either side of the larynx.

甲状腺峡
连接两个甲状腺叶的狭窄部分。

isthmus of the thyroid gland
Narrow part connecting the two lobes of the thyroid gland.

气管
肌性软骨通道。可使空气在喉和支气管之间通过。

trachea
Muscular cartilaginous channel allowing air to pass between the larynx and bronchi.

喉
肌性软骨通道。连接咽和气管，包含声带，具有发声和呼吸功能。

larynx
Muscular cartilaginous channel connecting the pharynx and trachea; it contains the vocal cords and has a vocalizing and respiratory function.

甲状旁腺
内分泌腺。位于甲状腺的后方，分泌的激素（甲状旁腺激素）可影响钙的代谢。

parathyroid gland
Each of the endocrine glands located behind the thyroid gland, secreting a hormone (parathyroid hormone) that acts on the calcium metabolism.

降钙素
甲状腺滤泡旁细胞分泌的激素。可降低血钙浓度，提高钙在骨骼中的浓度。

calcitonin
Hormone secreted by parafollicular cells, reducing the rate of calcium in the blood and increasing its concentration in the bones.

胶质
由蛋白质和碘组成的物质。位于甲状腺滤泡中，可储存甲状腺激素。

colloid
Substance contained in thyroid follicles, consisting of proteins and iodine and in which thyroid hormones are stored.

滤泡旁细胞
位于甲状腺滤泡基底部的细胞。可产生降钙素。

parafollicular cell
Cell located at the base of thyroid follicles, producing calcitonin.

滤泡细胞
围绕胶质的细胞。可产生甲状腺激素。

follicular cell
Cell surrounding the colloid and producing thyroid hormones.

甲状腺激素
甲状腺滤泡细胞分泌的激素。可加速新陈代谢，提高耗氧量和产热量。

thyroid hormones
Hormones secreted by follicular cells, speeding up metabolism and increasing oxygen consumption and heat production.

食管
肌膜性通道。构成消化道的上部，位于咽与胃之间。

esophagus
Muscular membranous channel forming the upper part of the digestive tract, between the pharynx and the stomach.

气管
肌性软骨通道。可使空气在喉和支气管之间通过。

trachea
Muscular cartilaginous channel allowing air to pass between the larynx and bronchi.

垂体

内分泌腺。受下丘脑调控。可分泌9种主要激素。这些激素主要针对生长、泌乳、血压和尿量调节等发挥作用。

pituitary gland

Endocrine gland that is controlled by the hypothalamus and that secretes nine major hormones that act especially on growth, lactation, blood pressure and urine retention.

垂体的结构
structure of the pituitary gland

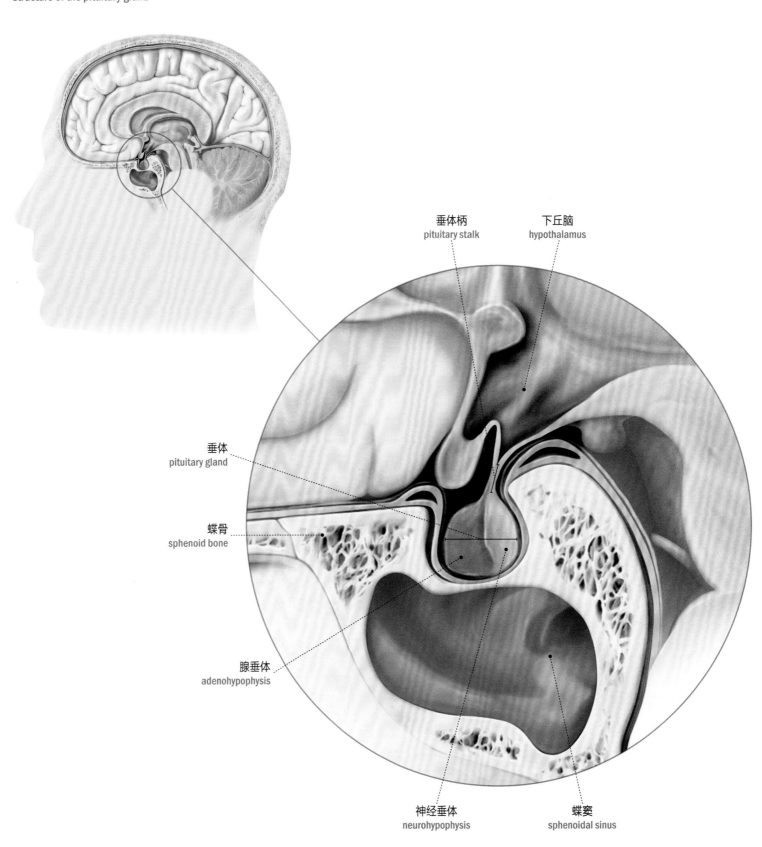

垂体柄
pituitary stalk

下丘脑
hypothalamus

垂体
pituitary gland

蝶骨
sphenoid bone

腺垂体
adenohypophysis

神经垂体
neurohypophysis

蝶窦
sphenoidal sinus

激素如何发挥作用 | Hormonal Activity

激素在血液中循环，遇到带有受体的靶细胞，即可附着于相应的受体。于是激素就可发挥作用，调节这些细胞的活动。有些反应会即刻发生，有些则需数日之后。

Hormones circulate in the blood and encounter target cells, which have receptors to which they attach. They then act on these cells by modifying their activity. The effects of their activity may be almost immediate or take a number of days to_appear.

垂体

内分泌腺。受下丘脑调控。可分泌9种主要激素。这些激素主要针对生长、泌乳、血压和尿量调节等发挥作用。

pituitary gland
Endocrine gland that is controlled by the hypothalamus and that secretes nine major hormones that act especially on growth, lactation, blood pressure and urine retention.

蝶骨

不成对的骨。位于眼眶后方，与头颅同宽。

sphenoid bone
Unpaired bone located behind the orbits and taking up the entire width of the skull.

腺垂体

垂体的前部。可分泌生长激素，也分泌对其它内分泌腺有调节作用的激素。

adenohypophysis
Anterior part of the hypophysis secreting growth hormone and hormones having a regulatory function on other endocrine glands.

垂体柄

富含神经元和血管的部位。将下丘脑连至垂体。

pituitary stalk
Area rich in neurons and blood vessels, connecting the hypothalamus to the hypophysis.

下丘脑

由灰质组成的小腺体。可调节垂体的激素分泌，控制自主神经系统活动。

hypothalamus
All the small formations of gray matter, controlling the hormonal secretions of the pituitary gland and the activity of the autonomic nervous system.

蝶窦

蝶骨的空腔。与鼻腔相通，可加热吸入的空气。

sphenoidal sinus
Cavity in the sphenoid bone, connecting with the nasal cavities and warming inhaled air.

神经垂体

垂体的后部。储存下丘脑神经元分泌的激素（血管加压素和催产素）。

neurohypophysis
Posterior part of the hypophysis storing the hormones (vasopressin and oxytocin) secreted by the neurons of the hypothalamus.

肾上腺 | suprarenal gland

肾上腺
内分泌腺。位于肾脏上方，可分泌多种激素，其中有的参与应激反应，有的调节水、盐代谢，维持电解质平衡。

suprarenal gland
Endocrine gland located above the kidney; some of the hormones it secretes are involved in the stress response while others act on water retention.

肾上腺剖面
section of a suprarenal gland

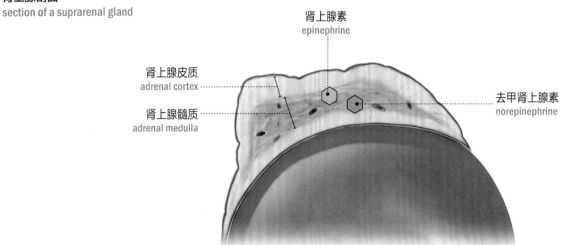

肾上腺素
epinephrine

肾上腺皮质
adrenal cortex

肾上腺髓质
adrenal medulla

去甲肾上腺素
norepinephrine

肾上腺皮质剖面
section of adrenal cortex

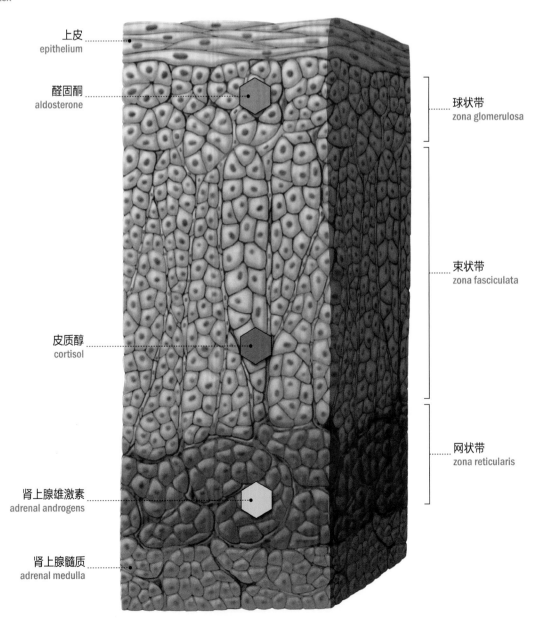

上皮
epithelium

醛固酮
aldosterone

皮质醇
cortisol

肾上腺雄激素
adrenal androgens

肾上腺髓质
adrenal medulla

球状带
zona glomerulosa

束状带
zona fasciculata

网状带
zona reticularis

肾上腺剖面

每个肾上腺都由两部分构成：肾上腺髓质和肾上腺皮质。这两部分均独立工作，并分泌不同的激素。

section of a suprarenal gland
Each surrenal gland is made up of two structures (medullosurrenal and corticosurrenal) functioning independently and secreting different hormones.

肾上腺皮质

肾上腺的外面部位。可分泌多种激素。

adrenal cortex
External part of the surrenal gland that secretes several hormones.

肾上腺髓质

肾上腺的中央部位。在应激状态下，可分泌肾上腺素和去甲肾上腺素。

adrenal medulla
Central part of the surrenal gland that secretes epinephrine and norepinephrine in stressful situations.

上皮

由致密上皮细胞构成的组织。具有覆盖、分泌和保护功能。

epithelium
Tissue formed of tightly knit epithelial cells that have covering, secretory and protective functions.

醛固酮

维持血液和组织液中钠钾平衡的激素。

aldosterone
Hormone maintaining the balance of sodium and potassium in the blood and interstitial fluid.

皮质醇

具有抗炎作用的激素。参与应激反应，可影响睡眠和食欲。

cortisol
Hormone having anti-inflammatory properties, intervening in the stress mechanism and affecting sleep and appetite.

肾上腺雄激素

激素。可促进毛发生长，为青春期做准备。

adrenal androgens
Hormones stimulating hair growth and preparing for puberty.

肾上腺髓质

肾上腺的中央部位。在应激状态下，可分泌肾上腺素和去甲肾上腺素。

adrenal medulla
Central part of the surrenal gland that secretes epinephrine and norepinephrine in stressful situations.

肾上腺素

在应激状态下分泌的激素。可使心率加快，肌肉里的血管扩张。

epinephrine
Hormone secreted in stressful situations, causing the heart rate to increase and blood vessels in the muscles to dilate.

去甲肾上腺素

可收缩血管，使血压升高的激素。

norepinephrine
Hormone causing blood vessels to contract and blood pressure to rise.

球状带

肾上腺皮质的最外层。可分泌醛固酮激素。

zona glomerulosa
Outermost layer of the corticosurrenal secreting aldosterone.

束状带

肾上腺皮质的中间层。可分泌皮质醇激素。

zona fasciculata
Middle layer of the corticosurrenal secreting especially cortisol.

网状带

肾上腺皮质的最内层。可分泌雄激素。

zona reticularis
Innermost layer of the corticosurrenal secreting androgens.

图书在版编目（CIP）数据

人体图典：奇妙身体说明书 / 加拿大 QA 国际原著；
王卫明，李箭主译 . —北京：人民卫生出版社，2022.8
书名原文：The Visual Dictionary of the Human
Body
ISBN 978-7-117-32508-0

Ⅰ.①人… Ⅱ.①加… ②王… ③李… Ⅲ.①人体解
剖学 – 图谱 Ⅳ.①R322-64

中国版本图书馆 CIP 数据核字（2021）第 240844 号

图字:01-2020-6778 号

人体图典：奇妙身体说明书

The Visual Dictionary of the Human Body

原　　著　[加]QA 国际
主　　译　王卫明　李　箭
出版发行　人民卫生出版社（中继线 010-59780011）
地　　址　北京市朝阳区潘家园南里 19 号
邮　　编　100021
印　　刷　北京华联印刷有限公司
经　　销　新华书店
开　　本　710×1000　1/8　　印张：27
字　　数　999 千字
版　　次　2022 年 8 月第 1 版
印　　次　2022 年 8 月第 1 次印刷
标准书号　ISBN 978-7-117-32508-0
定　　价　259.00 元

E – mail　pmph @ pmph.com
购书热线　010-59787592　010-59787584　010-65264830
打击盗版举报电话:010-59787491　　E – mail:WQ @ pmph.com
质量问题联系电话:010-59787234　　E – mail:zhiliang @ pmph.com